SAVING MY NECK

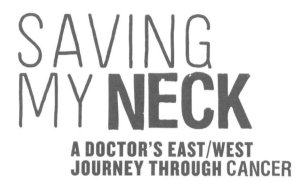

SAVING MY NECK

A DOCTOR'S EAST/WEST
JOURNEY THROUGH CANCER

TIMOTHY McCALL, MD

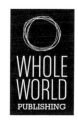

WHOLE
WORLD
PUBLISHING

4 Howard Street
Burlington, VT 05401

ISBN 978-1-7336521-0-0
Copyright ©2019 by Timothy McCall

FIRST EDITION

Cover painting by David Grotrian
www.davidgrotrian.com

Design by Gotham City Graphics
www.GothamCityGraphics.com

For Tony, the real scholar in the family

CONTENTS

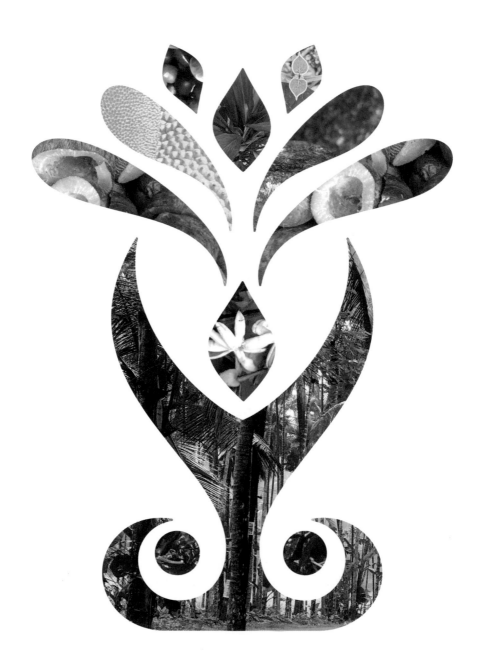

INTRODUCTION

In 1984, I began working as a doctor, first in a hospital as an intern and resident, and then in outpatient settings as a specialist in internal medicine. In 1997, after 13 years of practice, I quit and turned my attention to, of all things, yoga and yoga therapy. In late 2016, I was diagnosed with an oral squamous cell cancer that had spread to my lymph nodes. This turn of events forced me to return my focus to medicine — this time as a patient.

The human papillomavirus (HPV) — which causes several common cancers including the potentially deadly one that struck me — is the most widespread sexually transmitted organism in the world. It's estimated that 20 million people in the US harbor the virus, with more than six million new cases per year. Studies suggest that 80 percent or more of sexually active people who have not been vaccinated against it have been infected with the virus at some point in their lives. Those at risk include anyone who became sexually active before 2006 when the first HPV vaccine was introduced. In the vast majority of cases, the infection is cleared without treatment within a year or two.

Most likely, my immune system cleared the infection, too, though perhaps more slowly than most. But by the time that happened, the virus's DNA had already infiltrated mine. The infection is usually asymptomatic, as it was in me, which means I didn't know I had it and could have unwittingly passed it on to others. It's believed that the primary way the virus gets into the mouth is via oral sex, although open mouth kissing may be enough.

Some strains of HPV cause cancer. Others cause genital warts. Only rarely does the same strain cause both. This much has been known for some time. And there is a test — the Pap smear — that can detect changes in the cervix that precede the development of malignancy. In late 2017, the Pap smear was replaced by the Cervical Screening Test, a similar procedure, which includes a test for HPV. When the precursors of cervical cancer are detected, they can be removed before a malignancy has a chance to develop.

But there is no such test for the precursors of oral cancer like the one I had — which affects men about five times as often as women — and no way of knowing which people infected with the virus will end up with oral cancer. If you were infected at some point in the past, there's also no way to know if a small piece of HPV DNA is hiding somewhere in the DNA of a few of your cells, setting the stage for cancer. Nor was HPV's role in causing oral cancer understood when I was infected with the virus — likely decades ago, according to my doctors. This particular kind of cancer often takes many years to develop.

Only recently has the medical community become aware of an alarming increase in HPV-related oral cancer. In 2010, there were around 7,500 new cases of oropharyngeal cancer in men in the US. The number of new cases in 2018 was estimated at approximately 12,000 —

this despite a decline in cigarette smoking, which is a major risk factor for oral cancer. Epidemiologists expect the incidence of oropharyngeal cancer to continue climbing until 2030. The incidence in women is around 2,700 cases per year and is also climbing, though more slowly than in men. Growing majorities of these cases in both sexes are due to HPV.

Growing, because ever since the "sexual revolution" that began in the 1960s, it has become more common for people to start having sex earlier in life and to have multiple partners. Oral sex has become more common, too. There is evidence that smoking marijuana, which also became more common in the same period, increases the risk of HPV-related oral cancer. Not only is the number of cases increasing, but because there's no good screening test for such oral cancer, tumors tend to grow bigger and are more likely to metastasize before being detected.

The most common locations for HPV oral cancer are a tonsil, where mine appeared, and the back of the tongue. Usually by the time the cancer is found, it has already metastasized to lymph nodes in the neck — greatly worsening the prognosis. I spotted mine when it was an asymptomatic growth on my left tonsil no bigger than a dime — but by then it had already spread to three nodes on the opposite side of my neck.

None of my doctors could explain why my cancer crossed to the opposite side, since metastases usually appear on the same side. This further raised the risk that the treatment would fail. Another "negative prognostic factor," as doctors call it, was seen on my MRI. It looked like the cancer might have eaten through the outside capsules of one or two of my lymph nodes.

I have spent nearly 25 years studying yoga therapy and holistic healing, both in the United States and in

India. This includes many years of immersion in the ancient Indian holistic medical system called Ayurveda. In planning my cancer treatment, I chose to take an integrative approach. I wanted to take advantage of both the healing worlds I have inhabited, first as a western-trained doctor and then as a yoga therapist.

I was treated with chemotherapy and radiation, though I negotiated with my doctors and did not follow the proposed treatment plan in every detail. And because I was determined to use any means necessary to get better, I sometimes did other things that my doctors — who were excellent practitioners of conventional medicine — did not approve of (or wouldn't have, if I'd informed them). They were reluctant to recommend a treatment unless they had seen hard scientific evidence that it worked.

When you've got cancer, though, there isn't always time to wait for all the research to come in. You've got to evaluate the data, incomplete though it may be, and make the best choice you can. I was willing to try anything that my gut told me might help, as long as I felt sure that it was safe and wouldn't interfere with my conventional treatment. If it made me feel good, so much the better. If it was cheap and easy to use, better still. And if it made my chemoradiation easier to endure, sped up my recovery, and increased my chances for a cure, that was best of all.

Unfortunately, when it comes to integrative medicine, the world-class medical center where I was treated was way behind the times. That meant that in order to use the broader approach I had chosen, I had to figure out a lot on my own (with a little help from friends and colleagues).

In my first book, *Examining Your Doctor*, I advised readers to actively scrutinize every aspect of the care they were offered before they decided to go along with their doctors' recommendations — or not. As a patient, I did not always follow medical advice, but when I said no, I tried to do so in a respectful way. Of course, being a doctor myself, I could draw on years of medical training and practice. This allowed me to talk to my physicians in their own language. They treated me as a patient, but also as a colleague.

In the end, however, I was always the one who made the final decision. I believe every patient (who is able to) should exercise the same power. I was an active and decisive advocate for myself every step of the way, as exemplified in my very first conversation with my oncologist. She told me, "I want you to know that you have a vote" in all treatment decisions. My first thought on hearing this was, *No, you've got a vote. I've got a veto.* Of course, I didn't say that out loud.

Dealing with cancer is a challenge I never asked for. Just before I was diagnosed, I had a dark moment while teaching a yoga therapy workshop in Belgium. Suspecting the worst, I pleaded to be spared. I'm not sure whether this prayer was addressed to the universe or to God or what.

Yet looking back on the two years that have passed since my diagnosis, I am grateful. The journey through cancer has brought me benefits I would never have expected, both physical and emotional. If not for the cancer, some of these benefits might well never have come.

We yogis tend to believe that things happen for a reason. In my case, I had a lot to learn. About myself. About cancer. And about what really matters most to me.

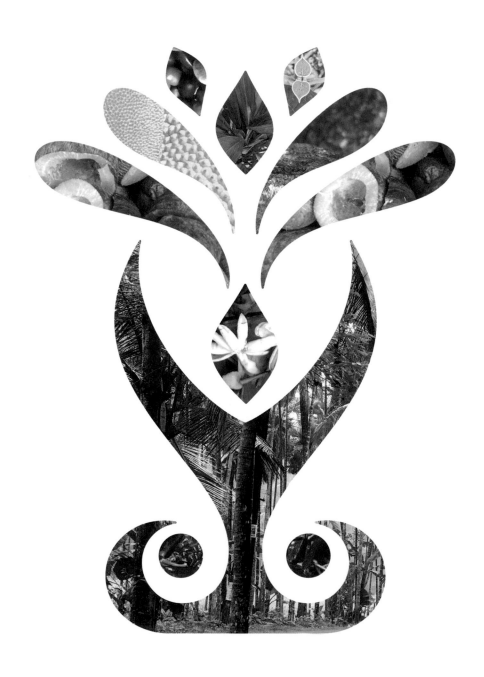

A NOTE TO READERS

This book is a memoir and is not intended as medical advice. Even though I've written books on health care for the public, *Saving My Neck* is not a how-to guide for dealing with cancer in general, or the particular kind that affected me. While I certainly hope my story will be of help to those facing cancer or other serious medical conditions, I am not suggesting anyone follow my exact approach. Indeed, most people in my situation should not, could not, or would not want to do all that I did. Though the diagnosis may be the same, the context in which it appears can never be. Another person facing the exact same disease might do better with a different overall plan than the one that worked for me. Please make all medical decisions in consultation with trusted health care professionals.

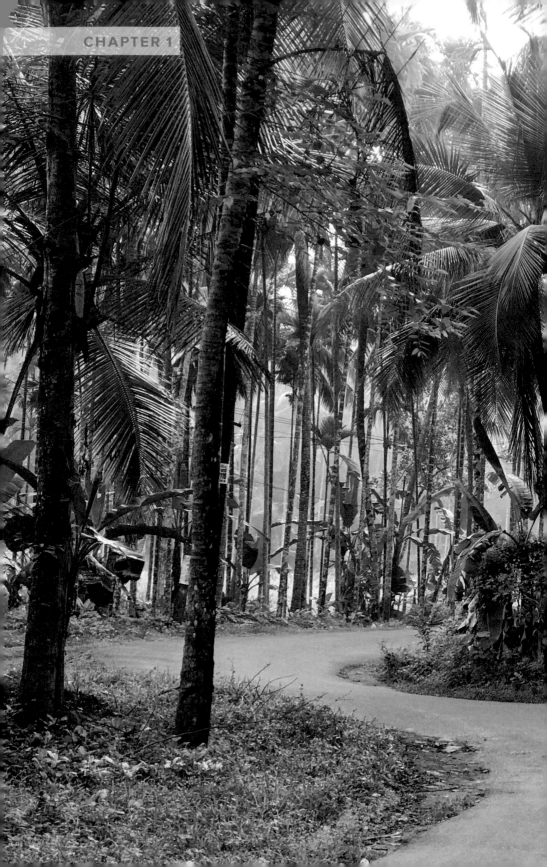

CHAPTER 1

"The part can never be well
unless the whole is well."

— Plato

SOME OF THE PARTS

Wearing only a muslin loincloth, I lie on a hardwood table. Its legs are still the original color, but the surface is stained dark from years of oil massages. A warm breeze stirs the sun-bleached crimson sari that separates the treatment room from the garden and the coconut palms outside. Krishna Dasan, the Ayurvedic therapist working on me, glides a warm, oil-infused bag in long firm strokes from my chest down the tops of my legs, and then back up. The bag is a handkerchief-sized square of cotton that has been stuffed with freshly-cut leaves, garlic, and lemon, and whose four corners have been tied into an elaborate knot which Krishna uses as a handle.

When he detects tightness in my body, Krishna moves back and forth over that spot with short staccato strokes, before resuming longer ones. When the bag cools, Krishna hands it to his assistant, Shashi, who puts it back into the turmeric-infused oil that bubbles on a single-burner gas flame, and hands Krishna a hot replacement. After pounding it once or twice on the table, to take the edge off the heat and remove excess oil, Krishna goes back to work on me. The air is fragrant with a smell more like food than medicine, something like homemade pea soup.

This is a treatment called Ela Kizhi, pronounced EE-lah KEE-ree. That means "leaf poultice" in Malayalam, the native tongue here in Kerala, the state at India's southwest tip. Systematically, Krishna massages my entire body, first with me lying on my back, then on my belly. Sometimes he has me turn onto my side with my top knee bent.

Though he isn't tall, Krishna is strong, with muscular shoulders and pecs. "I am never going to the gym," he says. He performs massage the way a dancer, martial artist, or yogi might. As he leans his torso to one side, he stays rooted in his feet, keeping him balanced. And although the massage is firm, the strength comes from his whole body and not just his arms.

When he was about nine years old, Krishna recalls, his father had about 100 banana trees. Krishna's assignment was to lug mud pots, each holding 20 liters of water, from the well to the trees. He estimates he walked five kilometers back and forth each day. The pots had no handles, so he would grip the inside edges of the rims with the fingers on either hand. As long as he was balanced, with one on each side, he was fine. This was when his muscles started to grow.

Because he is worried that the hot oil might cause the metastatic cancer cells in the lymph nodes of my neck to spread, he massages that area only lightly. A few days before we'd begun these treatments, his guru, the elderly Ayurvedic physician Chandukutty Vaidyar ("Vaidyar" being the Malayalam word for doctor), had warned him to be careful. Normally Chandukutty would not have approved of using Ayurvedic treatments for a condition like metastatic cancer, because he is not sure it can help. But I had been Chandukutty's student for years, so he made an exception for me. Krishna seems reassured when I explain that I am not expecting Ayurveda to cure my cancer — oropharyngeal squamous cell carcinoma caused by the human papillomavirus (HPV). I tell him, "I just want to get as rested and balanced as I can be before I undergo chemo and radiation treatments next month back in the States."

———————————

I hadn't expected to be able to come to India before my cancer treatment began. But the medical center where I would be getting my treatment was not in New York, where I was living at the time of my diagnosis, and my health insurance only covered treatment in my home state. So, I had to change my insurance, but it wouldn't take effect until after the first of the year. This meant I suddenly had a month free. On just a few days' notice, I planned this whole trip in late November of 2016 and arrived in India at the beginning of December.

In deciding to go to India for Ayurvedic care before beginning chemoradiation, I remembered something I had learned in medical school: cancer is potentially life-threatening, but in most circumstances, it is not an emergency. That's why I shudder when people hurry into treatments before they've had a chance to consider their options carefully.

The standard measure of cancer's growth rate is known as its "doubling time." For example, a slower-growing tumor might take eight months to go from one million cells to two million cells. Doubling every eight months would also mean it takes the same slower-growing tumor eight months to go from one cell to two cells, two cells to four, and four cells to eight. A rapidly growing tumor might double in size in 60 days. It's only at around a million cells — which roughly corresponds to one cubic centimeter in size — that tumors in some locations, like the breast, may be big enough to detect via X-rays or by touch.

It may take years, even decades, before a tumor is large enough to be detected. This is why a few weeks' delay — unless there is a critical situation like a tumor obstructing the breathing tube or compromising another vital structure — usually won't matter much. What's crucial to me is to get the best care possible, not, as I've heard patients say, to "get the cancer out of me as soon as possible." I had the luxury of not being in an emergency, so I was able to use the time to do extensive research, talk with loved ones, consult colleagues, get second opinions from other health care professionals, and come to India for Ayurvedic treatments — whose benefits I have been enjoying and studying for years.

It's around dinnertime on my first full day at Krishna's house in Kerala, a place I have been many times before. Krishna's phone rings. It's Chandukutty. He's across the paddy from the house. Krishna goes to fetch him.

Chandukutty greets me warmly when he arrives. "I am happy, very happy," he says, wrapping his hands around mine. He asks me to sit beside him and we exchange small talk. Our conversations are cordial, but for reasons I don't fully understand, they are never intimate. Maybe it's because his age, his culture, and his native tongue are all different from mine.

Bindu, Krishna's wife, serves Chandukutty rice and curry, while one of their daughters draws hot water upstairs so he can take a bucket bath. Krishna brings a fresh white dhoti for him to change into afterwards. Chandukutty has just been released from the hospital with, as best I can determine, the elderly equivalent of what in children is called "failure to thrive." Nonetheless, his gaze is strong and his skin is soft, moist and, except around his mouth and the corners of his eyes, unlined. Someone decades younger would be happy to have such youthful skin. This is the result of regular massages with healing oils for eight-and-a-half decades.

The three days Chandukutty spends at Krishna's house provide an unexpected opportunity for me to spend time with him. I'd called Krishna from the States to plan this trip and he'd informed Chandukutty of my diagnosis, so now I fill in some of the details for him. But part of me knows he doesn't need any of this information. Just laying eyes on me, he would have figured it all out.

In the years I've been with Chandukutty, I've repeatedly seen him show knowledge of things that no one has told him. When I first met him 12 years ago, he spotted my spinal condition in under a minute, even though all my medical-school professors, including orthopedists and rheumatologists as well as all my primary care physicians, had missed it. I myself had only learned of it three years earlier. Shadowing him as he evaluated new patients, time and again I saw him intuit the correct diagnosis for patients he had just met, whether it was back pain or diabetes or unspoken psychological problems, without an interview or physical exam. I have no idea how he does this.

Chandukutty loves taking the cases in which the conventional medical doctors have thrown up their hands, saying there's nothing more they can do. Nothing seemed to tickle him more than curing those people. The first week I shadowed him at his clinic, back in 2007, I saw him work some magic on a 20-something woman with sad eyes and a striking toothy smile. She had rheumatoid arthritis, a painfully destructive inflammatory joint disease. Despite high-dose Prednisone and methotrexate, big-gun western meds used to calm this autoimmune condition, she was bedridden.

Her family had carried her up the stairs to Chandukutty's clinic, which occupied a ward in an allopathic hospital in Calicut. At his direction, the female therapists gave her massages with medicated oils, infused with dozens of herbs. Herbal plasters were placed on her knees and other inflamed joints. Within one day, she was up walking with a cane. Within three days, she was walking without one. I sat in as he met with her during the second week of treatment.

Chandukutty asked her how much she was walking. She said half an hour a day. He told her he didn't believe her, but she insisted. Later that day, I checked with Krishna, who was at the clinic the whole time. He confirmed that she had not been telling the truth. Somehow, Chandukutty knew.

There is a way, though, that Chandukutty doesn't know how to teach me, and I don't know how to be his student. He understands how to raise a four-year-old to be like him. But he's not sure how to interact with an allopathic physician from another culture. I watch him carefully and ask questions, and I've learned tons from him, but none of it allows me to do what he does.

In Chandukutty Vaidyar's presence I get to witness Ayurveda as it's been practiced for hundreds if not thousands of years — undiluted — an experience not available in Ayurvedic medical colleges in the US or India. Everything he does is in the traditional way, except in cases where, say, a plant needed for a specific preparation is no longer available. Though he knows Ayurvedic theory, he is to his core a clinician. He sees the patient and he knows what to do, but can't necessarily explain it. I feel less like his protégé and more like one of those fortunate 20th century anthropologists who happened upon the last hunter-gatherer tribes unsullied by the modern world.

Chandukutty is a master of three different disciplines: Ayurveda; another ancient medical system called Siddha, from the neighboring state of Tamil Nadu; and Kalaripayattu, Kerala's indigenous martial art, which he practiced from early childhood. The last is said to be the historical precursor to Kung Fu and other Asian martial arts, first brought to the Shaolin temple by the monk Bodhidharma in either the 5th or 6th century. About a decade ago, Krishna tells me, a young thief tried to tear off Chandukutty's gold chain in a public bathroom. Chandukutty came down with his elbow on top of the man's head, knocking him out.

Back when Chandukutty was a boy, with the country under British control and Kerala ruled by the King of Malabar, there were no local police, and in most areas, no roads. Kalari masters were the de facto leaders. This didn't mean they had any more wealth than those they led — everyone was poor. The only cash was coconuts.

A few years ago, while I was staying at his house, I asked Chandukutty to demonstrate some Kalari. Despite his growing frailty, he moved quickly and gracefully, turning my wrist away with one hand and feigning blows to my torso with the other. I remember thinking: *This is a guy you would not want to mess with.*

I have been coming to India for 16 years, and in that time I have spent probably a couple of years here in total, most of it in this rural area along the coastal Malabar region of Kerala. The nearest city, Kozhikode, with half a million residents, is small by Indian standards, and off the tourist trail. Most locals still call it by the name the British used, Calicut.

If you've been to any of the large Indian cities, or even if you've just watched documentaries or read travelogues, you're familiar with the India of teeming metropolises, stunning colors in the markets, and air so polluted from auto fumes, industrial waste, and burning fields that it is dangerous just to breathe. You may conjure up visions of fabulous wealth and abject poverty side-by-side, shanty towns abutting gleaming high rises, shops and street food stalls emanating exotic smells, streets clogged with cars, auto-rickshaws, beggars, and skeletal cows that stop traffic. This place is nothing like that.

For one thing, it has so few tourists that every time I go for a stroll in the neighborhood, I am an event. School children stare at me with smiling eyes as they walk past. Men on motorbikes stop and offer rides. Children call out from houses: "Good morning" or "Where are you going?" Passengers on passing motorbikes and girls in matching uniforms, bunched together in auto-rickshaws, wave at me.

Some people — particularly older, more traditionally dressed folks — avert their eyes. But more common are greetings, usually in English. With a few people I have longer conversations. They ask, "What is your good name?" and "Which is your place?" I tell them and they smile and say, "Ah MAY rick ah."

Unlike other places I've been in this country, the prevalence of Christians in Kerala means that people usually aren't perplexed by biblical names like Timothy. Although it's been offered to me, I've never taken a Sanskrit name the way many western yogis do. But when asked, I sometimes say that the Indian people themselves have given me a spiritual name. Sometimes after

I've introduced myself, people have scrunched their faces, tipped their heads, and asked, "Trimurti?" After the first few times, deciding to go with the flow, I started to nod, "Yes, Trimurti." I'm told this is a most auspicious name. It signifies the trinity of three gods ("Murti" means god in Sanskrit), and refers to Hinduism's central male deities, Brahma, the creator; Vishnu, the sustainer; and Shiva, the destroyer.

Here, as in all of Kerala, the climate is semi-tropical. Abounding with inland waterways, it's lusher than most other areas of the country. Coconut palms and banana trees are everywhere. Houses are modest, often single-story structures made of bricks and mud, containing just a few rooms. Cows, chickens, goats, and sheep are as common as people. The air is clean. In recent years, concrete roofs have replaced thatched palm leaves, though the occasional house in Krishna's neighborhood has little more than a plastic tarp to keep out the rain.

By comparison with many of his neighbors, Krishna is doing well. Like many Keralite men seeking better pay, he spent several years as a young man working in the Middle East. With the money he sent home, his father and brother built this house. Five years ago, he was able to add a second floor, including a large indoor bathroom with western-style plumbing and two nice bedrooms, one of which I'm now staying in. As with the first floor, they built the addition on a shoestring, with a lot of sweat equity. A couple of years ago, they erected a corrugated steel roof, deeply pitched for monsoon rains, over an area of uncovered porch upstairs, which is now the treatment room.

More recently, Krishna's brother Manoj was able to build another house on the same land, which was divided among the two brothers and two sisters after their father's death. I've watched his house slowly take shape year by year. A concrete roof is in place but the red clay shingles haven't been laid yet. They sit, piled in rows in the yard, just as they were the last time I was here. They were bought used for a fraction of the cost of new ones. This was doubly smart since the old ones are of better quality than the ones now being sold. Even though the work on the house isn't finished, Manoj, his wife Poppi, and their two sons, Kanaan and Appu, have long since moved there from Krishna's place.

This area of Kerala has become a home away from home for me. I first stayed with Krishna and Bindu for a brief visit a dozen years ago. They've welcomed me back repeatedly since then, often for a month or two at a time. I've watched their three daughters grow up. Twenty-year-old Ashwadhi is already off at an Ayurvedic medical college in a neighboring state. This is an opportunity that even well-to-do women of previous generations didn't have — let alone those from poor families — and a big step up from the poverty that her father knew as a child. When Krishna was a boy, it took him two hours to walk the eight kilometers (five miles) uphill to school every morning. He often spent the day hungry, since his family couldn't afford to buy a midday meal. On a good day, as he walked home, he might find a coconut on the ground to snack on. Dinner was often kanji, a rice gruel, basically a way to stretch a small amount of grain. Or if he was lucky, they would have fish with tapioca, a starchy tuber that his father grew. Some days there was no food, especially in the spring once the year's tapioca had run out.

Krishna and Bindu's other two daughters, Aiswarya, the 17-year-old middle child, and Amrutha, the baby, are still at home with them and attending school. Aiswarya, now in her final year of secondary school, has announced that she's thinking of either studying Ayurveda like her sister or becoming a chartered accountant. The latter is a well-respected and well-paid job here, but somehow, it doesn't seem like a good fit for her.

Amrutha, now 14, is a tiny thing who only weighs about 60 pounds, but her personal power is palpable. Nobody has any idea what's going to become of this girl. Krishna has tried to steer her, but since she was a toddler, she's been impossible to control. She doesn't get into trouble but has a mind of her own. "Don't expect anything of me," she once told Krishna. He chuckles when he tells this story but says he doesn't know exactly what she meant, and hasn't asked.

———————

As I eat breakfast, Aiswarya stands behind Amrutha at the table and runs a curved-handle comb through her sister's hair, parting it in the middle. After poofing her sister's hair in the front, Aiswarya bends forward and brings her nose down to the top of Amrutha's head. A few minutes later as the styling continues, Ashwadhi, who is home on a brief break from college, walks into the room and brings her face to Amrutha's scalp. *What is going on?* Perhaps Amrutha had put some coconut oil in her hair, commonly done by women here, and her sisters are inhaling the pleasing aroma.

"Why did you smell her hair?" I ask.

"Yesterday I bought a packet of shampoo," Aiswarya says, "and I could smell it in her hair." Single serving pouches of detergent and shampoo, selling for a few rupees, are displayed on counter-top racks in local stores.

"No," Amrutha protests, "I didn't take a bath yesterday," implying that it couldn't possibly have been her who had pilfered the shampoo.

I look into Amrutha's mischievous eyes, remembering that they'd been to a Christmas party at the house of some Christian relatives the day before. "So, you are saying that you did not take a bath before going to your family's party? That's rude."

"No!!!" she steams.

Everyone laughs. Krishna tips his head and looks at her with love in his eyes and a smile on his face, which I take to mean *I think he's got you there.*

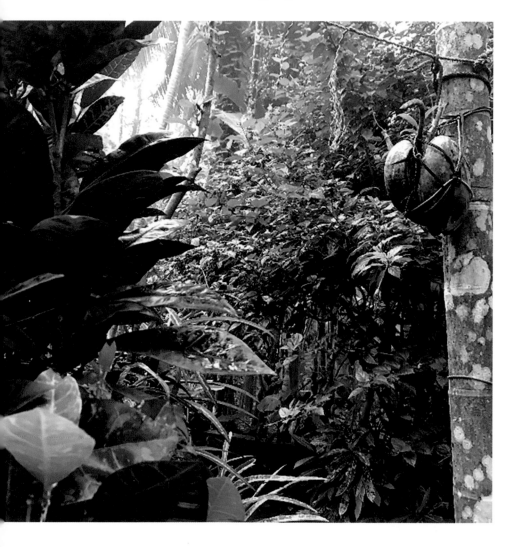

Although there is zero scientific evidence to support the idea, I have a hunch that the oil massages and herbal remedies that form the basis of the Ayurvedic treatments here might do more than simply balance and relax me. They might even increase my odds of getting cured. This hope isn't entirely crazy. It finds support in studies like those done by Dr. Raghavendra Rao and colleagues in association with Bangalore's Swami Vivekananda Yoga Research Foundation. The researchers found that when women with breast cancer added a gentle daily yoga practice to conventional medical treatments, they developed fewer side effects (fatigue, depression, anxiety, nausea, vomiting, etc.). When chemotherapy and radiation cause side effects that patients find hard to bear, oncologists often respond by reducing doses. Lower doses mean a greater chance that treatment will fail. For this reason, anything that lessens the side effects can increase the odds of a successful treatment. I didn't know for sure, but I was convinced that this Ayurvedic pre-treatment — a retreat in nature, where I could rest and practice loads of yoga — would reduce my side effects during chemoradiation. I remembered Chandukutty had said that the benefits of the oil massages continued to accrue for months afterward.

For most westerners, yoga is nothing more than the physical poses. But the breast cancer yoga program used in Dr. Raghavendra's studies added breathing exercises, chanting, and meditation, which are all components of traditional yoga. The women ate healthy vegetarian food and heard lectures on elements of yoga philosophy that are believed to foster healing. My teachers in India and in the States have taught me that yoga is a complete system whose components support each other. Even a short daily practice, if sustained for a long time, can be remarkably powerful. In a well-designed yoga practice, every aspect of body, mind, and spirit is addressed — this is the true meaning of "holistic."

The word "holism" is often misunderstood or used imprecisely. It does not mean natural, alternative, complementary, integrative, or spiritual — although holistic medicine might include approaches that fit any or all of these labels. Its main distinguishing characteristic is that it looks at the whole context — mind, body, and spirit, as well as environment, culture, and everything else that might affect a person.

As helpful as holistic measures can be, by themselves they may not be enough to cure some diseases for which modern medicine is more effective. Indeed, a recent study suggested that cancer patients who used only alternative treatments on average died sooner — and two-and-a-half times more often — than those who used both conventional and alternative approaches. This was true even though those who opted to employ only alternative therapies tended to be younger, more educated, and had higher incomes, all factors which would normally lead to better survival rates.

One aspect of the best holistic care, in my opinion, is that it welcomes treatments like drugs and surgery when they seem like they could help. From my experience as a practicing physician, however, I will say that aggressive chemotherapy and other cancer treatments are sometimes overused. For many malignancies, including mine, I believe the best results come from a combined approach. Such an approach takes full advantage of modern scientific medicine, while using holistic treatments to address the many areas of mind, body, and spirit that conventional medicine neglects.

Conventional medicine handles disease the way conventional agriculture handles crop pests: excise and poison the invaders until they've been killed off. Holistic medicine, on the other hand, resembles organic gardening: nurture the soil in which your plants grow, and your plants will be healthy. I'm using both of these approaches: the cancer is being dosed with toxic chemicals and radiation, while the soil of my body is cared for with healthy whole foods, deep relaxation and herbs.

———————————

Ayurveda is India's ancient holistic medical system. It's a natural complement to yoga, since both come out of the same philosophical system known as Sankya. The word Ayurveda can be translated as the "science of life" or "knowledge of longevity." For thousands of years, Ayurvedic doctors like Chandukutty Vaidyar have studied the effects of different foods, sleeping habits, climatic conditions, styles of exercise, and a host of other factors that contribute to, or harm, health and well-being.

I was initially skeptical of Ayurveda, which reminded me of ancient Greek medicine, but experience has won me over. Watching Chandukutty practice his medicine has also been persuasive. Now in his 80s, he is a living master, one of the last of a dying breed whose entire life has been dedicated to the pursuit of this discipline. In the evenings, he still reads ancient Ayurvedic texts.

Chandukutty is part of a long family lineage of Ayurvedic practitioners. His first exposure to Ayurveda would have come before he was even born. While she was pregnant, his mother would have received regular Ayurvedic massages, the oil and herbs making their way to her bloodstream and via the placenta to the fetus. She would have chanted Sanskrit mantras, the vibrations of which would have resonated through the amniotic fluid. After birth, he would have received daily massages and other Ayurvedic treatments. His apprenticeship with his father and grandfather began when he was still a toddler.

While I am still very much a believer in western medical science and chose to undergo conventional cancer treatment when I returned to the States, I can no longer look at health and healing without using the lens of Ayurveda. It is my hope and my belief that by adding its holistic perspective and its many tools, I may do more than just improve my chance of being cured. I may also be able to minimize the immediate side effects of radiation and chemotherapy, as well as some of the potential long-term aftereffects.

Ayurveda isn't the only holistic tool I've been using. Just after the cancer was diagnosed, days before I came to India, I had begun practicing chi gung visualization. I took the step on the advice of my medical school classmate, Srijan, a practicing family doc who's been studying this Chinese healing modality for decades. Several times per day, sitting with my eyes closed, I inhale and visualize that the tumor on my cancerous tonsil, and the three metastases on the other side of my neck, are burning brightly, flames rising from a white-hot core. Each time I exhale, I visualize gray smoke leaving my body, and the tumors glowing orange like fanned embers.

Although there is scientific evidence that visualization can work, I didn't look at any of it before I added the practice. I just figured the practice might help and couldn't hurt, so why not? I am surprised, though, that within days the tonsil, which pokes up half an inch above the back of my tongue, looks smaller, and the nodes that sit between the corner of my jaw and the collarbone feel smaller to the touch. In all my years of practicing medicine, I never saw a cancer shrink without medical treatments.

My Ayurvedic treatments appear to be having an effect, too. A few days after starting them, I notice that my tonsil is no longer covered with a grayish film, but is now shiny pink and looks even smaller in the mirror. When I move my fingers across the lymph nodes in my neck, as I've done thousands of times with patients, it feels like they are also shrinking. Krishna agrees. This trend continues over the next couple of weeks, with a palpable and visible decrease in the size of the tumors.

One brief interruption to the trend occurred halfway through my stay. Krishna and I had to travel by train to Kochi, five hours each way. That meant no massage, and a very long day. A hot one too, with Kochi's blazing noonday sun. Not ideal for an Ayurvedic patient — peak sun exposure should be avoided during treatment. The next morning Krishna and I noticed that the tonsil and nodes both appeared to have increased in size. After a few days of daily treatments and rest, they began to shrink again. I was amazed by how quickly the cancer seemed to respond to the changing conditions. And I felt encouraged to find that at least some of this appeared to be under my control. I had never expected that holistic treatment alone would suffice to eradicate the cancer, so I was still planning conventional cancer treatment upon my return to the States. Even so, these results told me that what I was doing had already made a difference.

So that you can understand the medical decisions I made, I need to explain more about the philosophy of holistic healing. Holistic healers don't diagnose and target specific diseases as conventional MDs do. They attempt to detoxify, strengthen, and balance the individual in ways that cause most medical conditions to improve. For example, in my yoga therapy work, I might use poses to improve a client's slumping posture, but not so much for esthetic reasons. Yoga teaches that poor posture can contribute to a host of ills: back pain, depression, carpal tunnel syndrome, and so on. If anxiety or insomnia is bothering the client, and if I notice that her breathing is choppy, I might teach her to slow and even out her breath. This can alter the balance of the sympathetic "fight or flight" and the parasympathetic "rest and digest" nervous systems, shifting her into a more restful, relaxed state.

It is because of this whole-person approach that holistically-minded healers are often more effective than conventional doctors in treating vague symptoms, undiagnosed conditions, and many chronic illnesses. And it is why adding holistic tools to the mix can both boost the effectiveness of conventional medical approaches and simultaneously lessen their side effects.

In conventional medicine, each diagnosis has its own treatment. Without a diagnosis, doctors don't know what to do. Symptomatic treatment may be possible, but that doesn't get at the underlying cause. In holistic medicine, it is the person that is treated, not the disease per se. This means that no western diagnosis is needed, and that treatment can always be given — even to those who are not sick, but who wish to improve their overall health and well-being.

Given the natural synergy between many holistic tools, combining several can make a big difference, and sometimes an enormous one. That's the way holism works. The more factors you align in the direction of better health and balance, the more a wide variety of symptoms — not just those related to the primary diagnosis — tend to lessen. Thus, to complement my conventional cancer care, I intended to use a multi-faceted approach, using as many tools as my time and energy allowed.

Yoga has been instrumental in helping me understand holistic health and healing; Ayurveda no less so. The yoga therapy work I do always incorporates an Ayurvedic point of view. This system, which dates back thousands of years, divides people and even animals into three major types based on observable characteristics, what scientists call phenotypes. Your genotype determines what your genes code for, and the phenotype is what results.

The three phenotypes, called doshas in Ayurveda, are vata, pitta, and kapha. Everyone has some mix of all three, and that mixture is their constitution, or "nature."

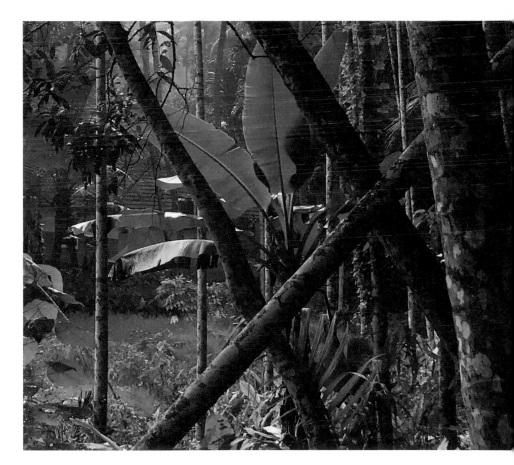

It is said that people in whom two out of the three doshas are about equally strong are more common than people with a single dominant dosha. People with all three in equal measure, so-called "tridoshics," are rarest of all.

Pittas, or fire types, tend to be intense, driven, and smart; they can be prone to frustration and anger, especially if they get out of balance. Ferocious tigers are a classic example. Pittas get inflammatory conditions like heart attacks, skin rashes, and ulcers. I remember seeing a photo of a three-year-old taken at Fenway Park, home of the Boston Red Sox, which captured pitta perfectly. Freckly, strawberry blond, his contorted face crimson with rage, the boy held his tiny middle finger high, saluting the ump who had just made a call that displeased him. Like increases like, according to Ayurveda, and a few hours in the sun-drenched bleachers would have stoked his fire. In Ayurvedic pulse examination, it is the middle finger with which the physician assesses the level of pitta.

In the Ayurvedic metaphor, kapha is made up of the elements of earth and water. People of this nature tend to be steady, stable, loving, and bigger-boned but, when imbalanced, prone to laziness, weight gain, and sadness. Elephants, said never to forget, typify kapha nature. Kaphas develop Type 2 diabetes and depression, and various diseases associated with swelling or excessive production of phlegm. Family and relationships are paramount to them. On pulse examination, Ayurvedic practitioners assess the level of this dosha with the finger that holds the wedding band.

Vata is like air and space. People of this constitution tend to be in constant motion, creative, enthusiastic, and, when imbalanced, impulsive and prone to anxiety. Animal examples are hummingbirds and bumblebees. Unlike pittas, with their sharply defined muscles, and kaphas with big, soft ones, people of vata nature, even if they lift weights, have trouble bulking up. They're susceptible to degenerative diseases of the joints and nervous system. Vatas are quick to understand and quick to forget, and their attention is easily distracted. The index finger, which like the mind can point in any direction, is used to assess vata in pulse diagnosis.

One day when I arrive in Krishna's treatment room, he and his brother Manoj, who resemble each other, are standing side by side.

"How come your hair is almost white and Manoj's is black?" I ask.

"This is the gift of my profession."

What Krishna means is that most of the treatments he administers, especially the hot ones like Ela Kizhi, warm the therapist's body. Ayurveda would say that the boiling oil is of the same nature as the fire of pitta, and would tend to increase that dosha. And pitta in Ayurvedic phenotyping is associated with premature graying.

If we were to liken the doshas to music, kaphas are the bass, vatas flutes and violins, and pittas an emphatic trumpet.

Rather than treating conditions like cancer directly, Ayurveda seeks to bring balance to the doshas. Doing so can help improve a wide variety of diseases and symptoms.

The opposite of holism is reductionism. Want to give a reductionism a try? Take any complex real-world phenomenon, and cut away everything except the one part you want to focus on. Most conventional medicine is built on this kind of thinking. That's true in the west and here in India as well, where "English medicine" now dominates. Reductionism also provides the theoretical underpinning for most modern science.

The idea is simple. Rather than looking at an entire organism, a reductionist studies the parts that comprise it. In medicine, for example, the heart is viewed as a collection of parts, each of which is studied in detail. Each of these parts is in turn broken down into its own constituent parts. In the case of the heart, reductionists examine the chambers, the valves, the coronary arteries, and every other part that can be identified. This process continues at ever-finer levels of organization, down to nuclei and mitochondria, hormones and neurotransmitters.

Reductionist thinking in medicine has saved millions of lives. Consider antibiotics, insulin, and the polio vaccine — even hand-washing. But, unfortunately, some physicians take a good thing too far. They put so much trust in the power of reductionism that they feel no need to consider the full humanity of their patients. When this attitude is taken to its extreme, the patient is seen as the sum of her lab tests and imaging studies. She becomes little more than a machine, some of whose parts can be fixed, others replaced.

The problem is that single-cause explanations of disease are oversimplifications. They contain truth, but they are not the whole truth. They fail to consider the whole context in which disease occurs — mind, body, spirit, and environment. Why do some people exposed to the same bug get sick, while others do not? Why do some victims of a disease survive years beyond the rosiest prognosis, while others are dead within months?

After a lifetime immersed in the field, I believe that we as a society have accepted a flawed understanding of health care. According to this understanding, there are two systems: modern medicine, and CAM (complementary and alternative medicine). The former is "real" medicine, grounded in hard data drawn from rigorous studies. The latter is fuzzy and unscientific, or so the claim goes.

Over the last 25 years, I've come to believe that this division of health care doesn't make sense. It is often arbitrary whether a treatment is placed on a pedestal as "scientific" or shunted to the sidelines as "unconventional." What's been accepted into the mainstream, and what hasn't, is as much a function of historical flukes, financial incentives, ideological biases, and intellectual blind spots as it is of truth or therapeutic effectiveness.

If an osteopathic physician adjusts your back, it's conventional medicine. If a chiropractor does it, it's CAM. You need a prescription for estrogen and insulin, but other human hormones, like melatonin and DHEA, are on the shelves in health food stores. Homeopathy was a much-respected part of conventional medicine in the 19th century; there were even homeopathic hospitals and medical schools across the United States, but then, in the early 20th century, the homeopaths were expelled from the AMA.

Some skeptics of CAM like to say that there are two types of medicine: one supported by evidence, and one not. By this standard, most surgeries for low back pain — which are not backed by randomized, controlled trials (RCTs), the so-called "gold standard" of proof — are alternative medicine. By the same standard, yoga, whose efficacy in treating back pain is now supported by more than a dozen RCTs, is conventional medicine. Try telling that to your insurance company.

If the lines are as blurred as these examples suggest, then perhaps we're asking the wrong questions. Maybe the whole CAM/scientific medicine divide is a red herring. Maybe there's something more basic that we're missing.

Around 1998, a year after I'd quit medicine, it started to dawn on me. The yoga that I was doing was healing me, but somehow it was doing it differently than the conventional medicine I knew so well. What made yoga so different?

Back then, I used to listen to a song called, "Love is the Drug." If my new love, yoga, was a drug, it was a gentler, slower-acting drug than the ones I knew. It didn't interact negatively with other treatments I used. Its side effects were sleeping better, having more energy, and feeling less back pain. The longer I did it, the stronger its effect. The drugs I'd prescribed, on the other hand, often became less effective over time.

Rather than attack a specific biochemical target, as drugs do, yoga addresses any number of factors simultaneously, nudging all of them towards health. When you do that — and especially when you keep doing that — the whole gets better. In contrast, with drugs, one factor moves in the desired direction, but, usually, other factors move in an unhealthy direction. That's what causes side effects.

Imagine that health is on a continuum, from −100 to +100, where zero represents nothing more than the absence of sickness. In conventional medicine, zero is the goal. Yoga aims much higher. No matter how healthy you are, you can always become healthier. That's what holistic healing aims for.

This, I realized, was the true divide: holism and reductionism. It's a fundamental philosophical difference. As an example, consider chelation therapy. It's a CAM treatment for heart disease, but in conventional medicine it's used in heavy metal poisoning. But no matter which category you put it in, the infusion of a synthetic chemical into a vein is reductionism. You're either aiming to affect a part, like a particular biochemical pathway, or you're aiming at strengthening and balancing the whole being. No amount of lobbying by interest groups can make a reductionist treatment holistic. A treatment is not going to be holistic this year, and reductionist two years down the road.

I also started to appreciate that holism isn't limited to alternative medicine. Good nursing is holistic. Conventional doctors who spend time getting to know their patients, and who use that information to inform the care they prescribe, are practicing more holistically. Perhaps the best example in modern medicine is hospice and other forms of palliative care. They employ a wide variety of measures — from the physical to the spiritual — to relieve the suffering of those facing serious illness or death.

Conversely, I realized that a high percentage of CAM practices are examples of what I now call "alternative reductionism." Consider vitamins. Even natural substances, benign when taken as food, can pose risks if concentrated and given in large amounts. For example, taking vitamin E pills has been found to raise the risk of lung cancer in smokers.

Some herbs that have been used safely in a holistic way for a long time can be harmful when a single component is extracted and used as a treatment — this is classic reductionism. Consider the herb *ma huang*, used safely in Chinese medicine for thousands of years. One of its ingredients, concentrated in pill form, became the supplement ephedra, which made headlines after it caused several deaths. Soon after, it was pulled from the market. The people who died from taking ephedra supplements were using enormous doses of these amphetamine-like pills — either to get high or to rev up their metabolism in an attempt to lose weight.

In general, whole herbs, used in a traditional way, are safe, whereas concentrated components in high doses should be approached with care. Failing to understand the difference between the safe, holistic use of *ma huang* and the dangerous use of its high-dose, reductionist spawn ephedra, US government officials issued a blanket restriction on both.

From what I've seen, little harm comes from traditional Ayurveda, Chinese medicine, bodywork, meditation, and other holistic approaches. I'm not saying no harm, but very low numbers considering the tens of millions of people who use them. Injuries may be common in strenuous yoga classes, but they're rare in yoga therapy, which is, by definition, tailored to the individual.

I suspect that the vast majority of the deaths and serious damage caused by CAM comes from alternative reductionist approaches. But because safer, and generally more effective, holistic approaches have been lumped into the same category as alternative reductionist ones, they suffer guilt by association. Another consequence of this dubious lumping together is that people who've benefitted from yoga and acupuncture and therapeutic bodywork often come to believe that "natural" vitamins and dietary supplements — even in huge doses — are more benign than they truly are.

My medical school professors talked about using chemical substances in "pharmacological doses." The implication was that it is the dose, not the substance itself, that makes a drug a drug. Although dietary supplements and mega-dose vitamins contain different chemicals than those in "drugs," the idea is the same: Find a target in the body and hit it with a biochemical hammer.

This is not to say that alternative reductionism has no place. It can bring benefits. Dietary supplements, even those with the potential to cause harm, appear to cause much less of it than drugs. Ephedra is estimated to have caused 17 deaths in the United States. In contrast, the

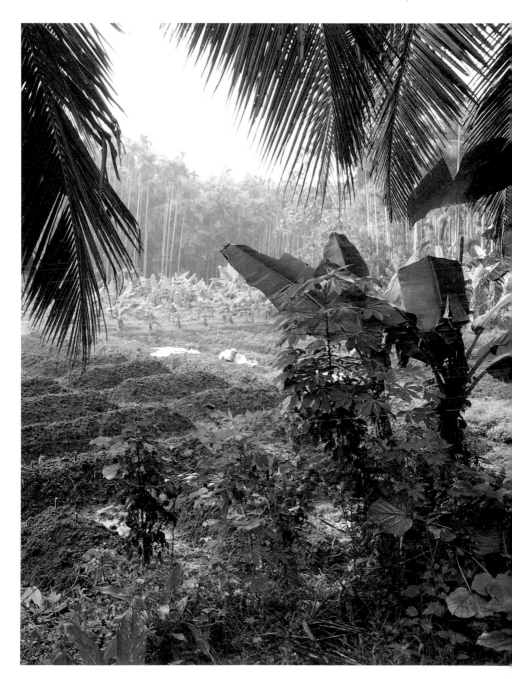

drug Vioxx is estimated to have caused 60,000 deaths. Still, reductionist approaches, including common alternative ones, cause more side effects than holistic approaches. They are also more likely to interact with other treatments, particularly other reductionist treatments. This is the reason that I generally frown on using too many alternative reductionist products at a time, or using a raft of them in combination with drug therapy. Nobody knows how they'll all interact.

That's why I hoped, as much as possible, to steer clear of alternative reductionist approaches during my cancer care. There's some evidence, for example, that antioxidant supplements can interfere with chemotherapy drugs, making the drugs less effective. If you're dealing with cancer, that kind of drug-supplement interaction could cost you your life. There are loads of cancer drugs, and an even greater number of possible combinations of cancer drugs. And there are hundreds of antioxidant supplements. Few of their potential interactions with chemotherapy have been studied, so nobody knows for sure how safe they are.

_____

Reductionist treatments typically act faster and, in the short-term, are often more effective than holistic approaches. But that changes over time: at first one pain pill works, then you need two; the antidepressant helps for a while, then doesn't. Reductionist treatments are generally cursed by diminishing returns; holistic approaches are blessed with ever-accumulating benefits.

The longer you take a pill, the more likely it is to lose effectiveness (there is one important exception to this rule: when you take just enough of a vitamin, mineral, or hormone to correct a deficiency, ongoing supplementation continues to work). When you attempt to change your body's biochemistry with drugs or supplements, the body adapts to compensate for any effects that it perceives as undesirable. When you take an antidepressant pill that raises serotonin level, the body responds by reducing the number of serotonin receptors — and that renders the same dose of the drug less effective over time.

Holistic treatments generally become more effective the longer you use them — slowly building like a savings account with compound interest. The idea is to change the organism from the inside out. Often, sustained effort is required, and learning is the outcome. Progress can continue for decades. In reductionism, by contrast, an outside force is used to change some aspect of your inner functioning: a drug lowers cholesterol levels, an angioplasty opens a blocked artery. All the heavy lifting is done for you — there's nothing to be done, nothing to be learned.

But that's not all. Holistic approaches are sometimes *more effective* than well-accepted, conventional reductionist medicine. Dr. Dean Ornish's program for heart disease is a perfect example. He employs a multi-pronged, holistic regimen that includes a whole-food, low-fat, vegetarian diet; smoking cessation; group meetings; exercise; and yoga, including poses, breathing exercises, and meditation.

The Ornish program has been shown to halt, and even reverse, blockages in coronary arteries. When Ornish's original study began in 1984, some subjects had chest pain and shortness of breath so severe that their doctors had recommended immediate bypass surgery. Yet without surgery — and without the statins and other cholesterol-lowering medications that many patients in the control group took — the patients' symptoms improved almost immediately, and they did better than the controls over the long haul.

Ornish's research also provides evidence that holistic approaches may help delay cellular aging, thereby increasing longevity. The ends of chromosomes contain what are known as telomeres. These DNA segments gradually shorten over the lifetime of the cell. When the telomere is reduced to a nub, the cell is unable to reproduce, and eventually dies. Ornish's program was able to achieve what no drug has ever been shown to do: increase the levels of the enzyme telomerase, which increases the length of telomeres.

More recently, Ornish has extended his program to men with prostate cancer. One study found that his regimen lowered prostate-specific antigen (PSA) levels, reflecting a reduction in the tumor size. The control group's PSA rose. The holistic approach also appeared to help the patients fight the cancer: their prostate-cancer cell growth was inhibited by 70 percent. In the control group, it was only nine percent.

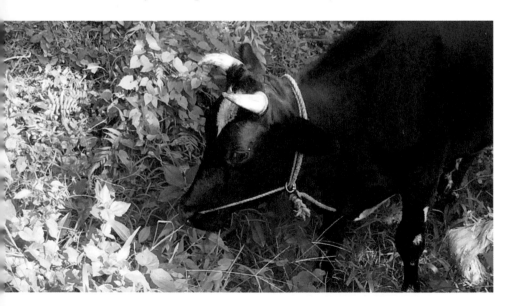

Another study, perhaps more relevant to my case, found that the Ornish program could cause changes in gene expression — this included a number of oncogenes (cancer-causing genes). Even if you have an oncogene, as long as it's in the "off" position, no harm can come from it. The participants had turned on hundreds of healthy genes, while simultaneously turning off dozens of cancer genes. No reductionist therapy has ever been shown to do that.

Drugs and surgery typically come out of the starting block faster than something like yoga or dietary changes. But a broad-based holistic approach can be the tortoise that wins the marathon of a long, healthy life. Yet despite all this evidence, conventional doctors continue to be skeptical of holistic healing.

Devastated by her unexpected defeat in the US presidential election, Hillary Clinton used a yoga breathing technique to help quell her anxiety. She happily demonstrated the practice, called "alternate nostril breathing," in an interview on the cable news station CNN as part of a book tour. Her claim caught the critical eye of James Hamblin, MD, a senior editor at the venerable *Atlantic*, who rejected it.

That alternate nostril breathing could actually have helped Clinton sounded impossible to Hamblin. "I tried breathing through only one nostril at a time," he wrote. "I couldn't do it." Then he figured out that Clinton used her fingers to alternately block each nostril. Hamblin wondered why the practice could possibly be calming. According to Hamblin, "Inducing partial suffocation isn't the most intuitive anti-anxiety ritual."

Hilary Clinton's claim that breathing through one

nostril stimulates the opposite hemisphere of the brain was ridiculed by Dr. Hamblin, mockery being one of the favorite tactics of conventional medical attacks on holistic healing. I've fought this my entire career in yoga. Too often doctors — as well as some health care journalists — look for the stupidest thing that's ever been said about some practice, and hold that up as evidence that the practice shouldn't be taken seriously.

Clinton had written in her book: "The way it's been explained to me, this allows oxygen to activate both the right side of the brain — which is the source of your creativity and imagination — and the left side — which controls reason and logic." Her explanation was mostly accurate, but she got one key detail wrong — the effects don't appear to be caused by oxygen.

Hamblin pounced. He gleefully responded that given the stress she was under, "she has more pressing concerns than considering how inhaled air goes down into the lungs, where oxygen is transferred to capillaries filled with blood that then go to the heart. The heart has a single left ventricle, and it shoots blood up to the head, oxygenating the brain's hemispheres with the same blood."

Hamblin dismissed the various "studies" cited by CNN, using scare quotes to emphasize their dubious nature. These trials had small numbers of participants, he complained, or were published in journals like The International Journal of Yoga, which, he wrote, "conceivably has some degree of pro-yoga bias."

Physicians criticizing holistic medical practices often have little knowledge or direct experience of the modalities they are discussing, yet they would like you to believe that, since they are scientists, they should be the arbiters of what works and what doesn't. If a practice sounds fanciful to a doctor, as alternate nostril breathing did to

Hamblin, then that's the end of the discussion. This is a phenomenon known as "proof by authority." Another way of saying this is, "Trust me, I'm a doctor."

Dr. Hamblin ended up writing off Clinton's experience with alternate nostril breathing as nothing more than a placebo response — that is, no more effective than a sugar pill. This is the favorite argument that skeptical physicians use to explain away any positive result from a treatment they doubt works. The attitude seems to be that because it can't possibly work, therefore it doesn't work, even when (as in this case) the available science suggests it does work.

It's not my aim to single out Dr. Hamblin here. It's just that his article is a typical example of the way medical experts seek to delegitimize holistic healing. Their arguments may seem persuasive to those who don't notice the bias and the faulty logic. In the pages that follow, I'll examine Dr. Hamblin's analysis from several angles. And, I should probably mention that I've got a personal stake in this discussion — I've done alternate nostril breathing daily for 18 years, and have found that it balances my nervous system and calms my mind. When I follow it with meditation, as I do every day, that meditation is more focused than it otherwise would be. And, over the years, alternate nostril breathing has gradually allowed me to bring much more air into the side of my nose blocked by a deviated septum.

Many holistic modalities like yoga therapy, osteopathic manipulative medicine, myofascial release, and craniosacral therapy were invented by masters who have spent many years refining their perceptive abilities. These treatments require heightened sensibilities on the part of the practitioner, too. And from what I've observed, these modalities can be even more powerful when the patients have also cultivated their inner awareness.

Many scientists have not cultivated their powers of perception, and when they investigate these modalities, they may come to incorrect conclusions. This is what I believe happened when Dr. Hamblin considered alternate nostril breathing. He analyzed it only by thinking about it, not by learning to do the practice correctly, trying it for a while, and then seeing what he thought. Rational thought is important, but it's not the only way to discern the truth. When divorced from embodied experience, it sometimes misleads.

Recently, a 30-year-old woman with a skin disease died after receiving treatment from a naturopathic physician. He had given her an intravenous infusion containing massive amounts of curcumin, a concentrated extract derived from turmeric. This use was not in line with traditional practice: rather than using the whole root of the plant, one of its components was used as a drug. Reductionism strikes again. The spice turmeric, commonly used in curry, has anti-inflammatory and anti-cancer properties, and may well be responsible for the low cancer rates here in India. It is safely consumed by hundreds of millions every day.

Real food is the ultimate example of holism; processed junk is pure reductionism. Although some scientists and nutritionists like to pretend that they know the "active ingredient" in carrots is beta-carotene, and in tomatoes is lycopene, these are at best partial truths. These two plant pigments are part of a large group known as carotenoids — powerful antioxidants that give fruits and

vegetables their vibrant colors. But every food that contains carotenoids also contains thousands of other con-
stituents, most of which have never even been identified,
much less studied. And the ways in which all these different chemicals interact with each other is beyond reductionist science's ability to fathom.

Doctors told us for years that antioxidants like beta-carotene, and vitamins C and E, might help prevent
heart disease and cancer. On that basis millions of people, including me, took them as supplements for years (I
stopped years ago — maybe I'm getting smarter as I age).
More recently, lycopene has been recommended to lower
the risk of prostate cancer.

But actually, what the studies had found was that people eating *diets* high in these chemicals had benefitted. In
other words, those who ate lots of marinara sauce were
judged to have consumed high quantities of lycopene. The
latter was then presumed to be responsible for the health
benefits observed. Controlled studies of such chemicals
in pill form aren't always conducted, but when they are,
they almost never confirm the benefits suggested by the
studies of people who eat the whole food.

As I sit on the edge of the treatment table awaiting
my massage, I tell Krishna how happy I am that we were
able to squeeze this trip in. I feel like I'm going back to
the States in much better shape. As we speak, Krishna
holds in his hand the bottle containing the fragrant oil
that he applies to my head at the beginning of most of my
treatments.

This high-quality translucent blue container is
familiar to me. It's the very same one that I brought to
India, how many years ago I don't remember. It originally

contained sesame oil. It's made of thicker plastic than the bottles found in India, and it has a snap-up nozzle that allows a more precise flow of oil. In richer countries, that bottle would have been thrown out or recycled years ago, but here everything is reused.

Krishna tips the container and pours a puddle of chartreuse liquid into the center of his cupped right hand. Then in a well-choreographed move, he lifts the hand to the crown of my head, turns it over, and places his palm on my scalp, not losing a drop along the way. As soon as I smell the oil, a wave of relaxation passes through me.

Because this fragrant oil, the smell of which I can never get enough of, has been poured on my head thousands of times, the relaxation is by now a conditioned habit. After spreading the oil around my scalp, he'll scrub the skin, creating heat. Then he'll work it around the backs of my ears as if he were massaging a dog.

This year, he's added a new technique: With the pad of his thumb, he scours the midline of my skull starting between my eyebrows and then all the way to the back of my head. I find it delectable. He slaps the top and sides of my head with flat hands, then for a couple of minutes taps my scalp with his fingertips, like the flourish Indian barbers use at the end of haircuts. He tops it off by bringing his fist down on his own hand placed on the crown of my head, with a loud clap. The blow is surprisingly hard, yet pleasant.

Then I lie back for the massage.

Afterwards, I retire to my upstairs bedroom to do my homework. I've brought dozens of scientific papers from the States on the treatment of oropharyngeal squamous cell carcinoma caused by the human papillomavirus (HPV). In them, I repeatedly come across a word I haven't heard since the waning days of the Vietnam war: de-escalation.

In my mind, I hear it in the baritone of CBS news anchor Walter Cronkite, whom my father watched every night, with its percussive first syllable: DEE-es-kah-lay-shun. In the papers I'm reading, the word refers to the practice of reducing doses of chemotherapy and/or radiation.

Why is de-escalation a trending term? Radiation and chemotherapy work as cancer treatments because they destroy cancerous tissue. Inevitably, non-cancerous tissues are also damaged. In the case of oral cancer, such tissues as the salivary glands, the thyroid, and the esophagus are in the line of fire. Patients with HPV oral cancer are often in their 50s, and otherwise healthy. If they are cured, they may have to endure aftereffects for the remaining decades of their lives: salivary glands may no longer work, leading to a persistently dry mouth; swallowing may be painful or difficult. Food may taste unappetizing. Doctors are experimenting with de-escalation in the hope of sparing patients some of these nasty aftereffects. I read a survey that reported that four out of five patients said they would accept a marginally lower cure rate if it meant fewer long-term symptoms. This is exactly how I feel.

De-escalation studies are underway, testing lower doses of radiation and chemotherapy to see if they can achieve similar cures rates, with better post-treatment quality of life. But there's a problem. Since the higher doses have become the standard of care, outside of a clinical trial like the ones I've been reading about, practicing oncologists are reluctant to prescribe anything less than the standard dose.

I am not going to let that stop me.

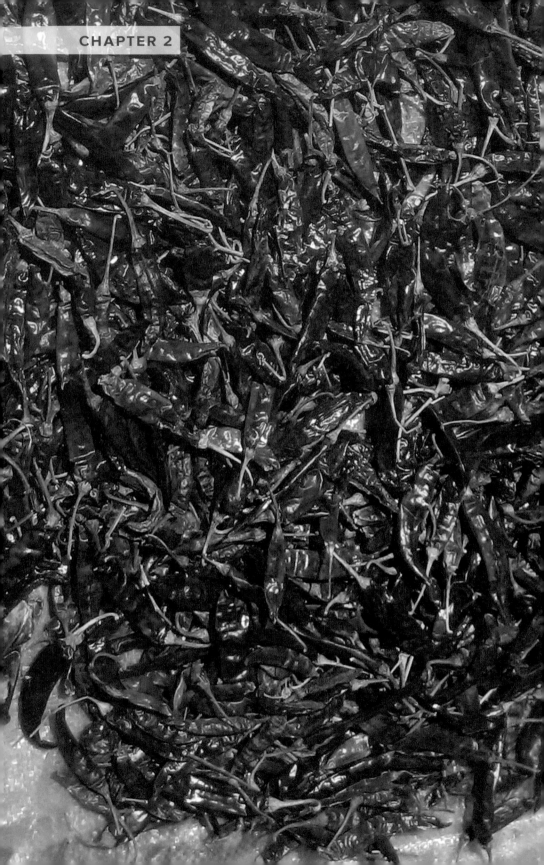

CHAPTER 2

"We can be absolutely certain only about things we do not understand."

— Eric Hoffer

EMINENCE-BASED MEDICINE

It takes me 24 hours to get from Kerala to JFK airport, but the journey isn't over yet. I then have an all-day drive south to my brother's house, where I'll be staying during my cancer treatment. I'm tired, but also pleasantly surprised that jet lag seems almost absent. The Ayurveda treatments are clearly working.

The next day, I go to meet Dr. Jeremiah Clark, the radiation oncologist who will be treating me (this and almost all of the health care professionals' names in this book are pseudonyms). I pull into the medical center's garage before I've even had a chance to fully unpack my car.

I have chosen this academic medical center primarily because of my big brother Tony, who is on the faculty. He's an endocrinologist and a professor of medicine who does a lot of NIH-funded research. When I was sorting through my options, my gut told me that this world-class institution, offering state-of-the-art conventional medical care, was the place to go. I figured that during my treatments I might be able to stay with Tony and his wife, Madelyn — empty-nesters who live a couple of miles from the cancer center — and they were generous enough to welcome me. Even before I arrived, I'd heard that Dr. Clark, who specializes in head and neck cancer, is a rising star in the field.

I enter the cancer center, which is being remodeled, and take the elevator to the radiation oncology department in the basement.

Dr. Clark's ruddy complexion and pleasant manner lead me to suspect he's a pitta-kapha, the Ayurvedic constitutional type that's been coming into my life with great frequency in recent years. He's soft-spoken, and his voice is higher-pitched than I expected. He seems shy and slightly awkward, but I get the sense that he's a good guy. His star may be rising, but he doesn't act like the cocky bulldogs I associate with the type.

My cancer, Dr. Clark tells me, is Stage IVa. This system of staging assigns values based on the severity of the cancer, ranging from zero to four, typically written in Roman numerals, with Stage IV being the most serious. When there are cancerous cells but they haven't invaded nearby tissues, it is Stage 0 — aka carcinoma in situ. Stage I refers to early disease. Stage IV means the cancer is advanced, while stages II and III are intermediate in severity. IVa cancers like mine are smaller than IVb tumors or have less extensive nodes.

Another way doctors have of describing cancers is via TMN staging, which stands for Tumor, Metastases, and Nodes. Technically, infiltrated nodes are also metastases, but separating them in this system allows doctors to differentiate nodes close to the primary tumor from metastases in the organs or distant tissues, which are more dangerous and more likely to kill the patient.

My TMN stage, according to Dr. Clark, is T1M0N2c. The T value varies from zero to four depending on the size of the primary tumor — my tonsil — and how much it's invaded neighboring tissues. Zero means no primary tumor can be found, which sometimes happens in oral cancers. My tonsil is about 15 millimeters, or about 5/8 of an inch. My doctors were surprised I'd found it when it was so small. I'd discovered it in the course of investigating why I had persistent tongue coating, a sign of imbalance as seen Ayurvedically.

The M value is either zero or one, depending on whether or not there is any evidence of far-flung spread. My value of zero means that there was no evidence of distant metastases in my body, based on the PET scan. This does not exclude the possibility that I already have distant metastases that were too small to detect at the time I was staged — so-called micro-metastases.

N values range from zero to three, depending on the number of positive nodes, as well as their size. The c was appended to my number two because my positive nodes were on the opposite, or contralateral, side of the body.

Dr. Clark recommends the standard, huge dose of radiation therapy. I'm skeptical about this. Worse, because my nodes are on the opposite side from the primary tumor, he wants to irradiate both sides of the neck, greatly increasing my risk of a permanently dry mouth and other side effects.

"I feel like HPV cancers have been grandfathered into a very aggressive treatment regimen that may not be optimal," I say. I've researched this, and feel strongly about it.

There are two different squamous cell carcinomas of the head and neck that look identical under the microscope. The cancer I've got is caused by the human papillomavirus (HPV). The other oral squamous cell cancer is caused by heavy use of tobacco, alcohol, or both. Until the last few years, no one realized these cancers were two separate diseases, but they are. The HPV tumors like mine tend to happen to people who are younger and healthier. They respond more readily to treatment and have a better prognosis. But since no one understood this until recently, doctors prescribed the same aggressive treatment with radiation and chemotherapy to both cancers — and they continue to do so.

Dr. Clark tells me the current recommendation is to give 70 Gray of radiation therapy (RT). To put this dose in perspective, the amount of radiation in one Gray is equivalent to that in 10,000 chest X-rays. Thus, they are recommending a dose equal to 700,000 chest films. Seven hundred thousand. That's typically given at a dose of two Gray, five days a week, for seven weeks. I am hoping to get a lower dose.

I tell him about a study I read in the oncology literature of a man with an HPV-related oral cancer who stopped at 46 Gray because he couldn't tolerate the side effects of RT — primarily the debilitating fatigue. Since his treatment was stopped early, his doctors had performed surgery to remove his primary tumor and the lymph nodes in his neck. When examined under the microscope, to everyone's surprise, all traces of the cancer were gone.

"I had a patient like that," Dr. Clark says, "who stopped after 30 Gray." In his case, too, when they operated, no evidence of the cancer could be found. "But I never wrote it up," he says, meaning he never submitted a report to a medical journal. He also tells me that back when he was a resident in radiation oncology, they treated people with tonsillar cancer with 60 Gray and they did well.

"Why don't we start treatment as if we are going to go to 70, and along the way we can decide," he says. As I'd planned my approach, I'd worried no one would honor my desire to use less than the standard dose. If they

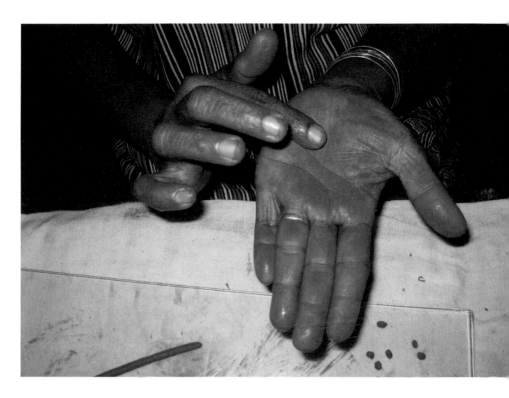

refused, I thought I might simply tell them when I got to the dose that seemed right that I was finished. But Dr. Clark, whatever his reservations, listened to me and acknowledged that I've thought this through.

"You're smart enough to figure out the right dose of radiation," Dr. Clark tells me.

"If you had to guess," I ask, "what dose of RT do you think you'll be using in five years?"

He says 66 Gray. I expected him to say something lower than that.

Dr. Clark provides an even more crucial piece of information. Each doctor I've talked to up till now has quoted 70 Gray as the recommended dose, but he says the guidelines actually call for 66 to 70 Gray.

Dr. Clark's willingness to work with me — to share information with me, to allow me to partner with him to figure out the best way forward — feels extraordinary to me. This is a doctor with whom I can speak my mind openly.

———————

I spent my first few days in town, between medical appointments, getting my living situation set up. How long exactly I'll need to stay here and when my treatments will begin remains to be seen. The treatments themselves may last six or seven weeks, depending on what I decide. Although the reasons for my being here are not good ones, this feels like where I am supposed to be. Not including the four weeks I just spent in India, and a similar trip the previous January after my wife and I split up, this will be the third place I've lived in the last year. I'd moved out of the home I'd shared with my wife, and strapped for cash I eventually found a room in a lovely house in the Hudson Valley of New York. That was the first time I'd had a roommate who wasn't a romantic partner in 30 years. Once I got my cancer diagnosis in November, and decided to come here, I'd packed up the remainder of my belongings and added to them to my storage unit in New York, and flew to India with no definite plans for where I was going to live after my treatment.

Here, however, Madelyn and Tony have done everything they can to make me feel at home. Madelyn has made space for my things in the dressers of my nephew Chris's old room, though his childhood storybooks and board games still line the shelves. Although it's a basement room, three windows allow good light and a view of the garden out front. I set up my laptop on the desk to help with my ongoing research of treatment options. And there's enough floor space for my yoga practice.

I brought a few houseplants in the car, and Madelyn lends me two giant palms with fat leaves, with which I line the windowsills. She even buys me a gorgeous Indian tapestry, floral with strong pinks and browns, which together we hang on the wall behind the bed.

One of my first purchases is a cool-mist humidifier. The winter air is arid and I've read that dryness of the mucous membranes that line the mouth and throat is one of the first treatment side effects to develop. The moist air should help, especially while I sleep. It should also benefit the plants. With the outside garden in the background, the room feels like a terrarium.

I'm very comfortable with this whole setup. But there is some possibility Tony and Madelyn will be moving soon. If so, I may need to move out soon after finishing treatments — perhaps around four months from now. Madelyn, a lawyer, has been interviewing for a big job as chief counsel at a college in the northeast. She doesn't want to get her hopes up, but I believe she will get it. For as long as I've known her, anytime she gets to the interview stage, she gets an offer. As impressive as her career looks on paper, it's her people skills that close the deal.

Madelyn has twice moved across the country for Tony's career, each time giving up great jobs and distancing herself from the community of friends they'd built. But this time, it would be Tony to make the sacrifice. He is close to retirement age and has accomplished a lot, culminating in his endowed chair at the medical school where I'm being treated. He is nervous about the prospect of figuring out what to do if they move but has committed to it if she lands the job.

Next up is a meeting with my medical oncologist, Dr. Melanie Shanahan, the person who will oversee my chemotherapy. While waiting in the examination room I hear a knock at the door, and in comes Dr. Shanahan's assistant, an oncology fellow named Dr. David Mitchell. He would have done a residency in internal medicine for three years, as I did, before starting a multi-year oncology fellowship. He looks young. His smile is warm and his manner casual. He reviews my history, asks a few questions and performs a brief physical exam, mostly of the mouth and neck.

As I expected, Dr. Mitchell encourages me to have Cisplatin alongside my radiation therapy. The chemotherapy, he tells me, is designed to make the RT more effective by weakening the cancer cells, not to be curative per se. Adding Cisplatin, he says, increases the effectiveness of the treatment by about 10 percent. "In this business, a 10 percent difference is huge."

Dr. Shanahan joins us. She's squat with a broad, handsome face and a ready smile. Early on, I ask her about a de-escalation trial I read about in India that compared high-dose Cisplatin, the standard treatment, given three times over the course of seven weeks, to a smaller dose infused weekly. The research found that the response rate was similar but the side effect profile for the lower dose was better.

Dr. Shanahan acknowledges the possibility of employing the smaller weekly dose, but favors the higher dose. She says there is better evidence of its effectiveness. She usually only recommends the smaller dose to people who might not be able to handle the larger dose; not someone like me who is strong and otherwise healthy.

I ask Dr. Shanahan to compare the side effects of the two dosing regimens. She maps out a comprehensive analysis of all the major risks of each option — in more detail than any physician I've ever seen. I feel grateful for that. There were three differences in the side effects she lists that I find significant. The higher dose increases the odds of developing kidney failure, which could necessitate life-long dialysis. There is a greater chance of nerve damage. It's also more likely to cause hearing loss.

I already have high-frequency hearing loss, well-earned from too many loud concerts as a younger man. I estimate I've attended more than 1,000: Big Joe Turner to Sarah Vaughan, Alison Krauss to Crowded House. My guess is I lost decibels of auditory acuity a single night at a Springsteen concert in Milwaukee. This was the first tour after the "big man," saxophonist Clarence Clemons, joined Bruce and the band. I stood stage-right, directly in front of a wall of speakers, to get a better look during a wailing sax solo on "Tenth Avenue Freeze-Out", and lingered far too long. My ears rang for days.

Although it doesn't affect me that much day-to-day, any additional loss of hearing caused by the chemo likely would. According to Ayurveda, I may also be more vulnerable to nervous system side effects given my life-long elevation in vata. That threat concerns me. The specter of dialysis, in particular, weighs heavy. One principle I use when making medical decisions is that a small chance of something really bad happening needs to be given extra weight.

"I want the low-dose weekly version," I say.

Dr. Shanahan, I think, is shocked. "If you change your mind," she says, speaking at a faster rate than earlier, "let us know as soon as possible so we can change the orders."

I know that won't be happening.

———————

Still recovering from the arduous journey from India, the long drive south, and my medical appointments, the afternoon of my second full day in town I come to my yoga practice. Seated in a forward bending pose, I am suddenly overwhelmed by fear — it arises spontaneously, and I have no idea from where. There's a constriction deep in my abdomen and a tightening in my neck and face. It arrives like a tropical storm on the ocean, waves crashing into the shore. What was buried beneath has been brought to the surface.

Unwelcome emotions sometimes arise during yoga practice. It's natural to want to do something about them, to change them in some way. I teach my students simply to let them be. I suggest they notice whatever arises — focusing on the physical sensations that accompany the emotion. This way, the sensations typically flow and ebb for a while and then the emotion abates. If you've ever tried to just observe an itch on your nose during mediation, without scratching it, you may have noticed that the itch gets more intense for a while, and then subsides. The same can happen with emotions.

The challenge is to stay with uncomfortable feelings, without getting wrapped up in the story that goes with them. If you can do that, I explain, the emotions often pass within minutes. Conversely, if you get drawn into the story — often a pattern of thought that may be all too familiar — the feelings tend to persist. While it's true that attending to the story can temporarily relieve painful feelings, chances are they will soon come roaring back.

I place myself into Child's pose, buttocks on my heels, torso folded forward over my thighs, my forehead resting on folded hands. What started as fear has now become terror. My heart thumps in my chest. My breath wants to speed up, too, but I keep it slow and smooth. Even though the physical sensations of fear are strong, I'm able to step back and observe them.

I have plenty to fear from the cancer and the impending

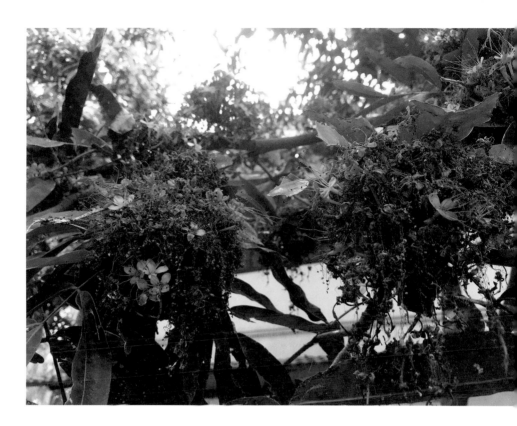

treatment. Perhaps in the constant activity these last two months — the trip to India, the Ayurvedic treatments, the intensive study of cancer, and the long trip home — I hadn't left room to feel the fear that must have been there all along. It seems that I haven't fully dealt with all the emotions I should have. It wouldn't be the first time.

But as I lie on my yoga mat, no story is attached to the fear, only raw sensation. This makes it easier for me to keep my focus on the bodily feelings as they go through their changes. The wrenching constriction persists. Each time the emotion lets up, I flow into another pose, or simply rest in Shavasana (Corpse pose) on my back, arms and legs splayed to the sides. Yet, again and again, the fear returns. It is exhausting to keep paying attention. This goes on for hours until I lose track of time.

Finally, the fear abates, not to return, the waves of emotion falling back into the sea.

――――――――――

Sitting alone in a windowless examination room, I wait nearly an hour for the ENT doc to appear, but I am fine with that. Dr. Peter Morrison is a busy man, and as a favor to Dr. Clark, he's made room for me in an already-overbooked schedule. I'm due to start radiation therapy and chemotherapy next week, and Dr. Clark thought I should see him before we began.

When Dr. Clark suggested the referral, I told him, "My gut feeling is that surgery isn't necessary." He nodded, and without quite saying it, I believe he indicated that this was his feeling as well. But in the case of an oral cancer like the one growing on my left tonsil, he wanted an ear, nose, and throat surgeon involved, in part because of institutional protocol.

When Dr. Morrison arrives, assistants in tow, I behold a fit, middle-aged man with thinning hair buzzed short and a neatly-trimmed goatee. He speaks animatedly, urging me to have the latest robotic surgery to remove the cancerous tonsil, as well a second procedure to take out all the lymph nodes from the front of both sides of my neck (not just the three on the right side that harbor metastases). His major selling point for the operation is not an increased chance for cure — there's no evidence for that — but rather that surgery would mean that I wouldn't need as much radiation therapy (RT).

"The side effects of the RT go up in a straight line with increasing dose," Dr. Morrison says. He describes in excruciating detail the dry mouth and intractable swallowing problems that often result from the recommended course of RT and chemo. I might be in for a life of not being able to enjoy food or get it down without difficulty and pain. The acidic state of the mouth from the absence of saliva, due to the destruction of the glands responsible for its production, could cause my teeth to rot — despite my best efforts at dental hygiene. Although I'd have long scars on both sides, he assures me that my neck would only end up about an inch thinner.

I ended up deciding against what I jokingly started calling a "bilateral modified radical neckectomy" (an allusion to the breast cancer treatment). But I absorbed Dr. Morrison's message about the potential side effects of what lay ahead — and for that I owe him a debt of gratitude. Despite all the reading and preparation I'd done, it was only after this visit that I understood in my bones what is at stake.

With a IVa cancer, more of my focus had been on saving my figurative neck — that is, on not dying. Only now, did I see that even if I survived, my literal neck would still need saving from the potential and devastating aftereffects of treatment. I'd had all the pieces of this puzzle for some time, but somehow I didn't see the whole picture until I heard Dr. Morrison's graphic and terrifying description. I immediately started looking for additional ways to minimize the damage.

I mention to Dr. Clark in our next meeting that I plan to take the lower weekly dose of Cisplatin. He says that his read of the literature is that it is the total dose, not the amount given at any one time, that seems to be the most important factor. If I take five weekly treatments, that would be the same amount of drug as two rounds of the higher dose regimen. I'm reassured to hear his opinion. Although my take from reading the studies was similar, he knows the research a lot better than I do. Dr. Morrison, on the other hand, had disparaged my choice of "the less effective dose."

Then Dr. Clark gives me a surprising piece of news: one third of patients getting the higher dose stop after two doses. They can't tolerate the final dose because of

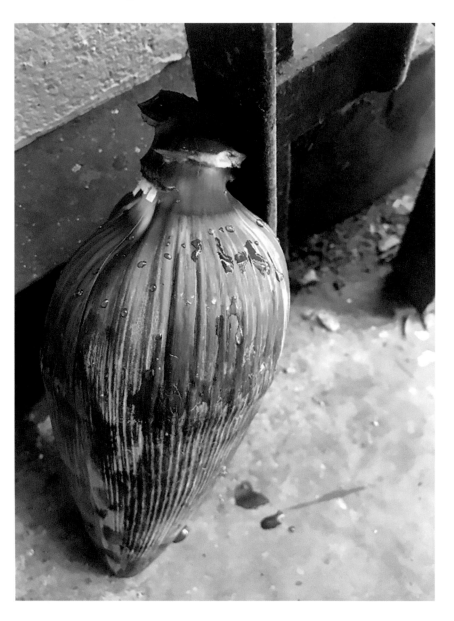

the side effects. I relay this to Dr. Shanahan in our next appointment, and she says that, actually, two out of three patients stop after the second dose. I'm surprised this information wasn't volunteered earlier, and I feel even surer of my choice to go with the lower, weekly dose of Cisplatin.

My second week down south, I meet my new primary care doctor, William Morley. He's the internist that Tony had suggested. Dr. Morley wonders whether I should have a zoster vaccine to prevent shingles prior to my treatments, but says he could go either way. I decide to think about it.

The painful skin rash of shingles — known medically as herpes zoster — only hits people who've had chicken-pox. The virus that causes both chicken pox and shingles lies dormant in the body after the chickenpox has cleared, sometimes for decades, hiding in a nerve root. Stress of various kinds can reactivate it, leading to an outbreak. Typically, you get blisters on one side of the body in the area of the skin that that nerve connects to. These crust over and can become extremely painful and, worse, the pain can persist long after the rash has cleared. Serious complications including widespread inflammation of the brain and blindness in an eye are also possible.

I sleep on it and decide to get the zoster vaccine. I am about to become immunosuppressed from cancer treat-ment, and if I were to get shingles then, it could be devas-tating. Influencing my decision is the funny relationship my immune system seems to have with the virus in ques-tion, varicella. Supposedly, you can only get chickenpox once — yet I had two documented cases as a kid. As an adult, I've had shingles three times. My most recent epi-sode about ten years ago was painful, but the first two were not.

Many members of the general public and many CAM practitioners are suspicious of vaccines. They believe that immunization causes side effects that aren't acknowledged by the medical establishment. I don't dismiss the claims of harm caused by vaccines. We are tinkering with the immune system, and there's no way there aren't going to be some serious side effects.

What vaccine opponents seem to miss, however, is how many lives vaccines have saved — numbering millions in my lifetime from the likes of polio, measles, and hepatitis. As with every medical decision, it's a matter of weighing the potential risks versus the benefits. Although I never considered a zoster vaccine before, given the specter of impending immunosuppression, it now seemed worth it.

I made a similar decision to vaccinate last fall. Days after getting diagnosed with cancer, I went to a local drug store with a friend to get a flu shot — which I hadn't done the year before. Beyond potentially benefitting me, I was aware that when I started my cancer treatment, I'd be around others who were immunosuppressed. By getting vaccinated when I did, I hoped to lower the odds that one of them would catch influenza from me.

––––––––––––

Sometimes, good scientific studies that might help guide your decisions are not available. This is the situation for nearly every holistic approach I'm considering. But for everything I am contemplating, there is at least some reason to believe it might help — and little apparent downside. Ruling out options because they aren't proven might mean never considering tools that might make a real difference, and maybe even save my life. My nutritional strategy is among those tools.

Leading up to my chemoradiation, I changed to mostly

vegan foods, what I call a "ghee-gan" diet. The only animal product I consume is ghee — clarified butter with all the milk solids removed. I have no doubt that ghee is deeply therapeutic for me, and it's really tasty. It's got no animal protein, which some evidence suggests may fuel cancer. I stop eating all other dairy products and eggs, worried by some of what I'm reading. Some observers suggest foods designed to promote rapid tissue growth in calves and embryos may induce the wrong kind of chemical signaling when you're trying to fight cancer.

Madelyn opposes my decision. Tony agrees with her, but doesn't say anything to me directly. They want me to build myself up and consider eggs and dairy products healthy foods — and they believe that my strategy is foolhardy. But wanting to do everything possible to improve the anti-cancer "terrain" in my body, I stick with my decision.

While unproven, I like the idea of potentially weakening the cancer via yet another mechanism — different from the other tools I'm using. Striking disease from many angles simultaneously is a cornerstone of holistic healing. It also happens to be a central strategy in conventional cancer care. That's why my doctors are planning chemotherapy and radiation simultaneously. My plan takes that strategy several steps further — by addressing some of the many aspects of health and healing that oncologists tend to neglect.

Since I know I might not be getting all the nutrition I need once side effects kick in, I'm ingesting as many high-nutrient foods as I can now. I brought my industrial-strength blender in the car for making smoothies a few times per week. I buy a masticating juicer, which extracts juice at lower speeds than other machines. From an Ayurvedic standpoint, its juice retains more of the fruit's essence — what yogis would call prana — as fewer cells are destroyed. You also get more juice, as the slower extraction process is more efficient. I figure that if I'm unable to eat solid food during my treatment, that I may be able to use the blender and juicer to ingest quality nutrients.

Most days, I'm making vegetable juices with a little fruit added for sweetness. I'm also imbibing smoothies, adding on different days ever-changing combinations of kale, chard, romaine lettuce, spirulina, chlorella, wheat grass, chia seeds, pumpkin seeds, hemp seed kernels, walnuts and pecans, cacao nibs, bananas, and berries. I've been making fresh almond milk out of nothing but pre-soaked almonds and water, blended and strained. It's silky and needs no sweetener and tastes as full of prana as fresh-baked bread. By comparison, the white liquid you find on grocery store shelves feels as pranically dead as those spongy sliced breads wrapped in cellophane. A friend of mine calls this kind of food "chi-free."

The common translation of prana is life energy — but when it comes to food, another way of expressing it is vitality. Fresh-squeezed orange juice — which my father served my mother every morning in bed — tastes more alive than reconstituted versions, even though nutritionists view them as the same. A fruit drink with high-fructose corn syrup and calcium added might be judged as nutritionally superior to the real food, because of the higher calcium levels.

When my mother was a girl spending summers on the family farm in Vermont, they'd put the water on the stove to boil, and only then go out to the field to pick the corn. That was because they could taste the difference between corn that was boiled within seconds of being brought back to the house and corn that had to wait 10 or 15 minutes for the water to come to a boil. The fresher the produce, the tastier and the higher its vitamin levels, too. But real food is a holistic entity whose effects can't be reduced to what little we know about its vitamin content.

———————

Tony and Madelyn's home has a large hot tub in the back yard. They keep the water hot enough that you need to wade in slowly. I've always been a fan of tubs with powerful jets for massaging yourself, and theirs gets deep into your back muscles. I'm surprised, though, that after a few days of indulging in the jets I find myself preferring to simply sit and soak.

Hyperthermia is an alternative cancer treatment I've learned about in my research. I read that even bringing the body temperature a few degrees higher than nor-mal, as happens in a fever, might be enough to make a therapeutic difference. Online I discovered that a few well-respected mainstream medical institutions offer hy-perthermia, believing it to improve the effectiveness of radiation therapy without increasing side effects. Those methods aren't available to me here, but my malignant lymph nodes run close to the surface, so I figure I might be able to heat them up by keeping my neck immersed in the hot tub.

It's hard to stay submerged enough to keep my neck under water. In the house I find a couple of 10-pound hand-held weights, which had been my nephew Chris's. I sit yoga-style on the bottom of the tub, holding a barbell in either hand. It's just enough weight to keep the water level at chin-height. My head is high enough to peer over the edge of the tub towards a row of pine trees and the golf course behind them.

I start out with just a few minutes at a time, but I work my way up to 30 minutes per session. I monitor my temperature with an oral thermometer, and am surprised that the reading reaches 102.9 F. The first few times at the longer durations, I felt dizzy afterwards and figured I'd gotten dehydrated. I began to drink large quantities of water before and after my immersions, and that solved the problem.

I add another piece to this practice, which might sound even more outlandish. It's said in yoga that chanting — which has a strong vibratory component — is potentiated if it's done in water. The ancient yogis probably had the Ganges in mind, but I figure it might be true in a hot tub, too, so why not? I chant a few Sanskrit mantras that are already part of my morning practice each session, feeling the vibrations in my head and neck, which are noticeably stronger than on dry land.

I admit, the notion that sitting in a hot tub chanting Sanskrit mantras might in any way affect the course of cancer sounds silly. But it's relaxing and softens my tight muscles. I'd lost range of motion in my leg in an injury last year. Ever since, I haven't been able to sit in my usual meditation pose on the floor. But in the hot water, I was surprised to discover I could sit cross-legged.

If it turns out that cancer cells are susceptible to the damaging effects of heat, the heat exposure could make a difference in the outcome. And if yoga's claims are correct about the healing powers of the specific mantras I've been using — not to mention the possibility that their efficacy increases in water — again I may benefit. Almost certainly, I'm not being harmed.

I have added a couple of minutes of chi gung shaking to my daily routine. To do this practice, you stand with your knees slightly bent, and without lifting your feet off the ground, repeatedly deepen your knee bend and come back up. This piston-like action sends a wave of movement throughout the body. To this, I often add a twisting action, though again my feet do not lift off the ground.

Many alternative healers recommend bouncing on a mini-trampoline to help increase circulation through the lymphatic system, an important element in the body's immune defenses. I suspect chi gung shaking has similar effects. But in my case, there's another motive.

I ruptured the tendon of the quadriceps, the large muscle in my thigh, just above the knee, during a hike last summer. In the weeks before the surgery, I was unable to use the leg much. For several weeks afterwards, I needed to wear a stiff knee brace that inhibited most movement of the leg. As a result, the muscle shrank to less than half its normal size. The shaking causes the quads to repeatedly fire, and that's part of my plan to rehabilitate the muscle.

Even though cancer is my main concern, all the treatment choices I'm making are affected by whatever else is going on with me. That's holistic healing.

———————

Although my oncologist Dr. Shanahan isn't interested in what I'm doing with the hot tub, Dr. Mitchell, her assistant, is. "Are you still raising your core temperature in the hot tub?" he asks. He seems amused when I tell him I have been.

Before Dr. Shanahan joins us, I show Dr. Mitchell a list I printed out that has all the herbs and other measures I plan to employ. While I was in India, I read an integrative oncology textbook cover-to-cover and consulted other resources, and I only opted for treatments that should not interfere with my conventional cancer care.

I've decided to mix herbs, medicinal mushrooms, and other natural elements — all in small quantities — into melted ghee, which I take by mouth. One Ayurvedic herb I'd had good luck with in the past is Ashwagandha, which is said to calm the nervous system, strengthen the body, and build immunity. To this I add Astragalus,

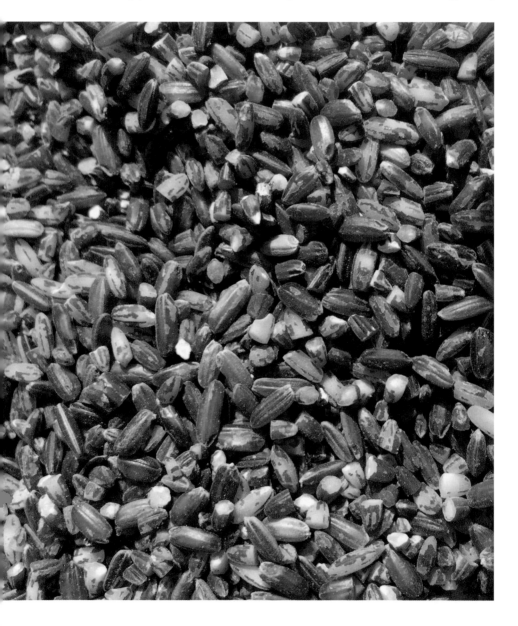

an immune booster from the world of Chinese medicine. Green tea has anti-HPV properties, so I add a pinch of deep-green matcha powder to the mix. Black raspberries have also been found to fight the virus, so I add some freeze-dried powder. I include my old standby turmeric, because of its anti-inflammatory and anti-cancer characteristics. I add various powdered medicinal mushrooms (Shiitake, Maitake, Turkey Tail, etc.), known immune boosters. Finally, I grind a few black peppercorns, grown on one of Manoj's trees in Kerala. Studies show that pepper increases the amount of turmeric absorbed by the intestines 20-fold.

I swallow a couple of teaspoonfuls of this mixture twice a day, a bit at a time, so as to be sure to experience its complex, bittersweet taste — as Ayurveda recommends. My plan is to continue these once the chemoradiation begins. Dr. Mitchell writes it all down and says he'll talk with the pharmacist to make sure everything would be safe. They look fine to him, he says, except for ginseng, which I've been considering adding but haven't purchased yet. He isn't sure about that one.

But after Dr. Shanahan arrives, she puts the kibosh on the whole plan. "Eat whatever you want, but I don't want you taking any of this," she says. Her smile is sweet but her tone is uncompromising. When my primary care doctor had recommended her in an email he sent me in India, he said she was young but highly respected within the institution. When I had asked if she was open to integrative approaches, he said he didn't know.

Dr. Shanahan had told me at our first visit that I had "a vote" in all treatment decisions. I knew her intentions were good, but it felt patronizing to me.

And now, I figure, she's rejecting my carefully-formulated plan out of ignorance. She's trying to protect me, but she doesn't know enough about integrative approaches to understand that I've done my homework and erred on the side of caution. This is another instance of a specialist telling a patient — even a patient who is himself a doctor — "Trust me, I'm a doctor." At this moment, I decide that she has the lost the right to be fully informed of what I am doing.

———————

I'm a believer in what you might call healing synergy. When different approaches are combined, their benefits add up to more than the sum of the parts. Synergy, I teach my students, is like $1 + 1 + 1 = 10$. Many holistic approaches are based on it.

Let's say you try 20 different tinctures, balms and massages, spend more time in nature, and keep a journal to explore your feelings. Some of these may turn out to be ineffective, but as long as they're safe, you haven't lost much. In my case, if even just a few of the unproven tools I'm employing end up contributing to the effectiveness of my chemoradiation treatment, reduce its side effects, or reduce its aftereffects, I will have gained a lot.

But the vast majority of physicians — all my doctors, as well as Dr. Hamblin, who had ridiculed alternate nostril breathing as a treatment for anxiety — follow the tenets of evidence-based medicine. EBM is currently the dominant ideology in modern health care. EBM believes that a doctor's clinical decisions should be based only on the available scientific evidence, not on opinion, intuition, or personal experience.

EBM advocates are sometimes dismissive when patients opt for unproven treatments. For the sake of supposed scientific purity, they would prefer that patients do without treatments that don't meet their standards. My question is: who's crazy here? These ideologues, or people whose lives are at stake who are willing to think outside the box, especially in those cases where nothing inside the box offers much hope? Or what about in a case like mine, where the conventional treatments do offer hope, but hope that comes at a high price?

Am I supposed to wait around till modern medicine decides it approves of approaches that I already can tell are helping me? EBM insists on proof of the effectiveness of any treatment *for each disease* for which it's used. While there are studies suggesting benefits of yoga for people with more than 100 health conditions, the cancer I have is not one of them.

There's no quackery here. No one is taking advantage of me. Nobody is profiteering off my suffering. There's no shunning of proven treatments to pursue dubious approaches at some clinic in Mexico. I'm a rational, well-educated physician who's done a boatload of research. I'm making clinical decisions that strike me as eminently logical and sensible. If my doctors don't agree, that's their problem.

"Is there any way we can shield the parotids?" I ask Dr. Clark. These half-dollar size salivary glands that sit behind either sideburn are in the RT's firing line, and I am hoping to find a way to mitigate the damage.

He is non-committal.

I ask him if the tonsil and nodes get 70 Gray, how much would the parotids get? He estimates 30 Gray. The research I'm reading suggests that if both sides get that dose, there is a serious risk of life-long mouth dryness.

"I don't want to die in order to avoid having a dry mouth for the rest of my life," I tell him, but I do want to minimize the dose as much as possible. Then I quote Dr. Morrison's statement that the side effects go up in a straight line with increased dose.

"Cure," Dr. Clark says, "also goes up in a straight line."

What I didn't realize at the time of our initial conversation is that Dr. Clark has the ability with the tomographic radiation therapy machine to deliver radiation circumferentially around the neck from any angle. He can choose which vectors to use, sparing selected tissues to some degree, as long as the targeted areas get the necessary dose.

Tomographic RT combines the now-standard intensity-modulated radiation therapy (IMRT) with computed tomography (CT) scanning. IMRT is a more accurate way to deliver radiation than older technologies, and can be more precisely directed to hit the tumor with less bombardment of neighboring healthy tissues, and the additional of tomography likely makes it even better.

With the "tomo" machine, a low-radiation CT scan is done before beginning each treatment. This provides a 3-D image, which allows the technician to assess the exact position and size of the tumor that day, allowing further precision in targeting.

I had heard there is an affiliated radiation facility closer to Tony and Madelyn's home, which might be more convenient for me. I ask Dr. Clark whether it would make sense for me to go there instead.

The problem, he says, is that the other location doesn't have a tomographic machine. "Can I tell you we see better results here? No, I can't." But he still thinks it would be better to stay. I decide to follow his advice.

"What about my thyroid?" I ask. This is another gland that my research indicates could be imperiled by the chemoradiation, and I realize we've never discussed it.

One thing I've learned about Dr. Clark, who I believe is an extraordinary physician, is that he will tell you about side effects if you ask, but if you don't ask, he will stay mostly silent on the topic. Without prompting him, there aren't a lot of warnings about what to expect.

"We can't protect everything," he says. "If we knock it out, we'll replace it."

He is speaking to me as one would with a medical colleague, and I understand what he means. If I develop hypothyroidism as a side effect of the treatments, they would prescribe thyroid hormone to bring my blood levels back to normal. It occurs to me that Dr. Clark, brilliant as he is, probably has no idea how bad this remark would sound to the part of me that is also his patient.

———————

The week before I'm due to start chemoradiation, I learn of research that suggests that acupuncture may be useful in improving salivary flow in patients undergoing treatment for head and neck cancer. I phone a community clinic, which offers low cost acupuncture. They keep the price more affordable by treating several patients simultaneously in a large room. I tell the receptionist my story and she puts me through to an acupuncturist who she thinks might be perfect.

The acupuncturist, who I'll call Martha, is a two-time cancer survivor as well as a registered nurse. I like what I hear, but I'm concerned that the group setting may prevent her from doing the kind of in-depth holistic evaluation that I hope will precede, and guide, my care. It is possible to speak for a few minutes in the hallway prior to entering the treatment room, she says, but we decided it would be best if I see her in her private office. There, she can spend the time needed to do a careful intake interview. She fits me in for the following Monday, two days before my chemoradiation is set to start.

In the lovely upstairs office of a converted neighborhood home, Martha and I talk for a long time. After feeling my pulse, she treats me with needles as well as moxibustion — the burning of herbs just above the surface of the skin over acupuncture points. When we finish, we formulate a plan. Thursday, the day after my first infusion of chemotherapy, I'll see her at the community clinic. She suggests I start coming Friday evenings to the town's health center for auricular acupuncture, in which five tiny needles are inserted into each of the ears. It's free, though donations are encouraged. And we've decided, I'll see her weekly in her private office. Our idea is to maintain this three-times-per-week schedule throughout my cancer treatment, and as long into my rehabilitation period as we deem appropriate.

A crucial element of evidence-based medicine is the insistence that all treatments must be justified by the same high quality research. This was the criterion Dr. Hamblin used to dismiss alternate nostril breathing. Yogis have known for millennia — and science has confirmed — that during most of the day, the breath flows preferentially through one nostril or the other. After some minutes or hours, the flow switches to the other nostril. This is known as the "nasal cycle."

Research by Dr. David Shannahoff-Khalsa of the University of California San Diego shows that breathing through the left nostril stimulates the right hemisphere of the brain, and vice versa. More oxygen doesn't cause the activation of the opposite side of the brain. The nervous system does that. But there is some truth in the left brain/right brain difference that Clinton described. This study, and another by the same author, examined the link between hemisphere dominance and the nasal cycle. Both were published in *The International Journal of Neuroscience*, which admittedly could have a pro-neuroscience bias.

There is also evidence that right nostril breathing stimulates the sympathetic nervous system's (SNS) "fight or flight response," while left nostril breathing is linked to the parasympathetic nervous system's (PNS) "rest and digest" response. Alternate nostril breathing might thus help balance these two branches of the autonomic nervous system, thereby relieving a condition like anxiety, which is associated with dominance of the SNS over the PNS. Likely even more important, the slow breathing and mindfulness required for the practice tends to be calming to both the nervous system and the mind.

Dismissing the studies cited by CNN, Dr. Hamblin arbitrarily decided that for him to be willing to consider the evidence, each trial had to have at least 50 participants. Such studies can cost tens of thousands of dollars to conduct. And because holistic interventions tend to work more slowly than drugs and other reductionist approaches, it might be necessary to do even more expensive, longer-term research to demonstrate any benefit.

What Hamblin failed to consider is that this is not a level playing field. Most research these days is paid for by the drug companies and other corporations manufacturing the products they are hoping to sell. This is different from the way things worked when I was in medical school, when the National Institutes of Health and other governmental agencies funded most studies. For something like yoga, there is no industry to sponsor research, and no patentable product whose profits might pay for it.

The yoga studies that are conducted often depend on the work of volunteers.

EBM's idea is that something like yoga therapy — which when skillfully implemented is extremely safe (and as far as we know has never caused a single death) — requires the same level of proof as pharmaceuticals, which kill tens of thousands of patients every year. This is not science — it's simply an idea about how science should be applied to modern medicine. And it's an idea that needs to be challenged.

———————

A few days before my treatment begins, I come across some research online that causes me to rethink my plans. A scientist named Dr. Valter Longo from the University of Southern California has been studying the effects of fasting on mice that had been implanted with various cancers and then treated with radiation and/or chemotherapy. Compared to mice that received normal rations of mouse food, rodents given only water for 48–60 hours during treatment were cured at higher rates, lived longer, and suffered fewer side effects. In some cases, fasting animals were able to tolerate doses of chemotherapy that killed the normally-fed mice.

As Longo explains, fasting causes a change in normal cells: they go into famine mode. Our ancestors faced periodic shortages of food, and as a result, they evolved adaptations that allowed them to tolerate fasting. And not just tolerate: these adaptations promote health in a variety of ways. One of them, as it turns out, is that the cells of fasting animals are less susceptible to damage from chemotherapy and radiation. Cancer cells, on the other hand, lack these adaptations, and don't do well without a constant supply of energy.

Doctors are generally reluctant to recommend treatment based on animal studies, but no good human studies have been done, and I don't have time to wait. Since no one profits when a patient fasts — except maybe the patient — such studies may never be done. I'm aware that spiritual traditions from around the world have prescribed fasting for millennia and, except for the elderly or seriously ill, it is generally well-tolerated.

Continuing my research, I come across more information about fasting by cancer patients. In an oncology journal, I find a report of dozens of patients with a variety of cancers who fasted before their treatments. One of the most striking results is that most of the patients experienced little or no nausea from chemo. This is very encouraging, because I have learned that Cisplatin, the drug I'll be on, causes such severe nausea that cancer patients call it "Cisflatten."

Dr. Shanahan is so worried about the potential for intractable vomiting that she's prescribed me three different anti-emetic drugs. Both she and the nurse manager assigned to my case have lectured me about "anticipatory nausea." This dreaded side effect happens when the first infusion of chemo causes nausea and vomiting so horrible that when it's time for the next infusion, the patient starts retching at the door of the clinic. The next time, it might start even earlier, perhaps during the car ride there.

On Tuesday, the day before my first chemo, I drink only warm water and don't plan to eat again until Thursday morning. That means 63 hours without any food. Until now, the longest I've ever succeeded at water-only fasting is one day. Will I be able to make it that long?

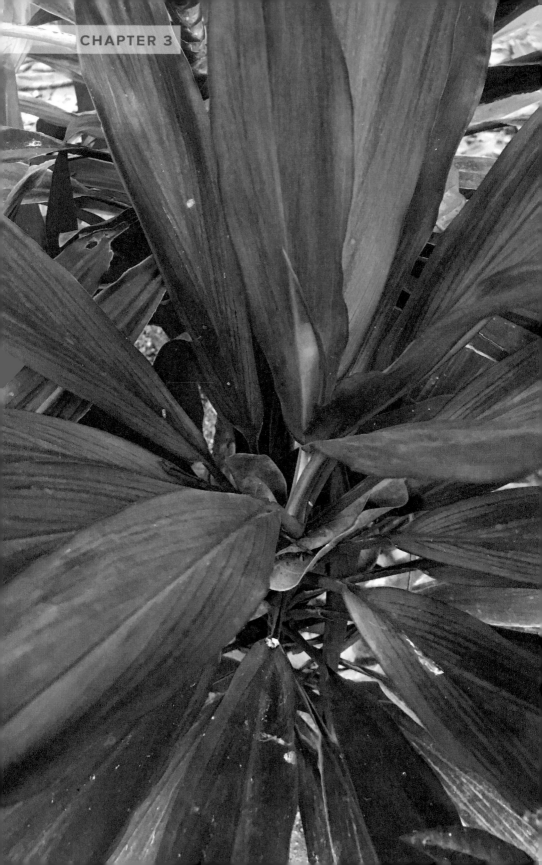

CHAPTER 3

"When the diet is wrong, medicine is of no use.
When the diet is right, medicine is unnecessary."

— Charaka

STARVING MY CANCER

For most of my life, I had no interest in fasting. If a meal was more than an hour later than expected, I'd develop a headache or stomach pain. If I ate within an hour of these warning signs appearing, the symptoms would abate. Any later than that and they would last for hours.

After I took up yoga, things changed. The practice is supposed to be done on an empty stomach. With classes scheduled at different times, I noticed myself developing more flexibility.

Three years ago, I tried fasting for a few days as part of an at-home Ayurvedic detoxification program. It did not go well. In this particular cleanse, you eat only kitchari, an Indian porridge made from rice and split mung beans. After the first day, I felt hungry and irritable, and despite my hunger it was hard for me to down much of the gruel — I craved something, anything, more interesting to eat.

But if fasting before my chemotherapy will reduce side effects and, more importantly, boost my chances of a cure, I'm willing to give it a shot. Another benefit of fasting is that it promotes autophagy, which is Greek for "self-eating." A large proportion of the energy the body expends in a day is used for digestion. When there's no food to be digested, that energy can be used to clean house — the body eliminates tired old immune cells and stimulates the production of new immunological stem cells to replace them. Dr. Yoshinori Ohsumi was awarded the 2016 Nobel Prize for his discovery of fasting-induced autophagy.

How long should I fast for each infusion? Researching online, I find no consensus. Many suggest three or four days, but that's probably too long for me. All oral radiation patients lose a lot of weight. Dr. Clark's nurse estimates the average at ten percent of body weight. Even before beginning, I am leaner than most.

If I had been willing to receive the higher dose of Cisplatin, it would have meant only three infusions over the seven-week course of treatment. Since I've chosen a lower dose, I'll be given an infusion every week, which means I'll have to fast every week. Three or four days of fasting every seven days seems like too much. If I get too skinny, my immune system could be compromised. Fasting may be healthy, but emaciation is not. I come up with a plan that feels like the best balance between feasibility and effectiveness.

My first chemo is scheduled for Wednesday afternoon. I eat a full meal at lunch on Monday, followed by freshly-pressed vegetable juice that evening. From this point on, I will ingest only water, until Thursday morning when I'll break my fast with another juice. During the fast, I won't even take my herbs. This schedule will mean about 63 hours of nothing but water, with a juice-fast transition before and after.

On Wednesday morning, I'm happy to discover that I don't feel that hungry and my energy is the about same as usual. I head to the cancer center for my first session of radiation therapy, followed in the afternoon by the first infusion of chemotherapy.

The air conditioning in the cancer center is freezing. I'm wearing a maroon stocking cap, one of several that Madelyn bought for me on an outing last weekend. Before the Cisplatin is infused, the nurse brings a paper cup with two pills. One is Decadron, a powerful corticosteroid, in this case being prescribed to reduce nausea. The other is a popular new anti-nausea agent that is said to be much more effective than the drugs that came before it.

Dr. Shanahan had wanted to prescribe 16 milligrams (mg) of Decadron, which I thought was too much. This drug is six times more powerful than Prednisone — I prescribed that powerful steroid a lot when I practiced medicine. Because of all of Prednisone's side effects, including agitation and immunosuppression, I avoided it whenever I could — and tried to use as low a dose as possible when I couldn't. I convinced her to try 8mg instead, still a hefty dose.

I have decided that I'm not going to tell Dr. Shanahan or my other physicians that I'm fasting. I'm still hopeful it will reduce the nausea and vomiting, which I've been dreading. It just makes sense to me that fasting could work: When the stomach is empty, the likelihood of nausea will be less. Many animals fast instinctively when they are ill.

In India, I've used this strategy to good effect when I've felt an intestinal infection coming on, marked by the familiar stomach cramps and sulphur-tinged burps. I'd simply stop eating for 12-24 hours, drink lots of fluids, and for good measure take a few acidophilus capsules. I have used this strategy multiple times to successfully abort impending gastrointestinal hell.

Just in case, though, I bring some preventive medicine for nausea. Sitting in the infusion center, I chew on an Ayurvedic herbal remedy: slices of fresh ginger that I've brought from home. Their tang is intense, but I've come to enjoy it.

As the yellow contents of the small bag of Cisplatin drip into a larger bag of saline that runs into a vein in my arm, I do not think of it as a toxic drug — though I know full well that it is. Instead, I imagine that it is a healing nectar flowing into me and circulating throughout my body. I lie back on the vinyl Barcalounger and look out the window at the few trees in this urban landscape while I silently chant mantras.

Since nobody knows what kind of shape I'll be in once I'm finished here, Tony has agreed to pick me up. I text him after 6 p.m. to say that I should be done soon. I don't mention that I could have driven myself. I'm not noticing any side effects at all.

That evening when it's time for bed, I am having palpitations like never before in my life. I'm convinced they're from the Decadron. It feels like I've drunk 10 cups of espresso, and I'm still flying after midnight. I finally get about five hours of sleep, not terrible, but not ideal at a time when you'd like your immune system to be at its best. I can only imagine what would have happened if they'd given me the full 16 milligrams.

I email Dr. Shanahan in the morning. She agrees — it's probably the steroid. She suggests we cut the dose to 4mg the following week and, if all goes well, we can discontinue it entirely. I'd rather skip it before next week's chemo, too, and see how I do that way, but I decide it's better to choose my battles. I let it go.

The next day, I go in for the second of my five-times-a-week radiation therapy sessions. I lie back on the platform of the tomographic RT machine. The technician straps me in and asks me if I would like a warm blanket. He returns with a heavy, piping-hot one, which he lays over my body. This becomes my favorite part of every treatment. Then comes my least favorite part: he places a plastic mesh mask, form-fitted the week before, snugly over my face — and bolts its edges to the platform.

From the booth, the technician asks me if I am ready. The platform slides into the tube in the middle of the large white machine. It whirs and clicks as he shoots the initial CT, the one he uses to target where he'll direct the radiation. The platform slides back out and I wait. After several minutes, it slides me back in. This time it's for the treatment, which lasts somewhere between five and ten minutes. It's noisy but I don't pay too much attention. As I lie in the machine, I silently chant yogic mantras. The techs had asked if I wanted the radio on but I said no. As with the chemotherapy and RT yesterday, I feel nothing during the treatment.

Early in my second week of treatment, I get an idea. I ask if they can move my Thursday midday RT appointment up to first thing in the morning, before I eat breakfast. That would mean that three out my five weekly RT sessions would occur while I'm fasting — instead of just two — potentially boosting the effectiveness of the treatment. They are able to accommodate my request, and no one asks why.

After being full of energy the during first three days of

my treatment — probably aided by the Decadron — Saturday morning, fatigue envelops me like fog. Dr. Shanahan had warned this might happen. I feel too weak to meditate sitting up, so I try it lying in bed, with marginal success.

Once I start chemotherapy, I stop setting an alarm to wake up. I simply allow my body to tell me how much sleep it needs. I don't want to impose anything on it — unless I have an early appointment. I'm averaging 10, 11, or more hours of deep sleep every night. I get up to pee because I am pushing fluids, even during the night, but I always fall right back to sleep.

When I first came to yoga, I had a huge problem with insomnia. When I was a medical resident, it was even worse. With all overnight shifts disrupting my sleep rhythms, I was taking a lot of sleeping pills. By about five years into yoga, long since off the medication, the insomnia was mostly gone. I never did any yoga designed to improve it. I just practiced, and my sleep improved.

The second round of chemo goes well. Once I again I have no nausea. I'm still chewing on fresh ginger, but may not need to going forward. I take the lower dose of Decadron, and at this dose I'm able to sleep better. My weight, though, is down about 3.5 pounds from when I started. My mouth is a little dry, a treatment side effect they warned me could arrive early. But the tonsil looks about half the size it was when we started — and the lymph nodes have also all gotten smaller. Dr. Shanahan agrees that the tumors have shrunk.

Tony and Madelyn do not support my decision to fast before chemo. Tony refers to it as "starving yourself." But my decision feels sound to me, and I have no intention of budging. I know they love me, and they believe I am making a mistake. There is no way to please them, and do what I feel I need to do.

Even though it's speculative, I am convinced it was the fasting that allowed me to get through my first two sessions of chemotherapy with no nausea or vomiting. If I need to eat food during future treatments, I am prepared to do so. But I breezed through the first two rounds, and figure I can handle four more fasts over the next month.

Early in my second week of treatment, I get a strong intuitive sense that I should reintroduce eggs to my diet. Soft-boiled eggs were one of my few childhood comfort foods. We ate them with salt and buttered toast cut into bite-size squares.

I decide to go with my intuition, even though some of my research suggests eggs may have a pro-cancer effect. You could make yourself crazy with this stuff — some doctor or nutritionist online will say negative things about virtually any food. If you followed all the advice you read, there wouldn't be anything left to eat.

In addition to the herbs I am taking, I'm also employing an Ayurvedic practice called "oil pulling." I take a sip of medicated oil — a few herbs in a mixture of sesame and coconut oils — and swish it around my mouth for 10-20 minutes. When I'm done, I spit the oil into the garbage. Ayurveda says that this practice removes toxicity from the body, but I'm thinking that it may also be good to bathe the oral tissues in the healing blend. For good measure, I add a pinch of green tea, turmeric, and powdered berries to the oil. I start doing oil pulling a couple of times a day, often while I read.

I get an email from Krishna — Chandukutty Vaidyar has died. It happened the day after my second chemotherapy infusion. I am sad that he is gone, but thankful for our years together. I feel especially grateful that I got to see him one last time so soon before he passed.

Krishna and I learned a lot from him, but tragically Chandukutty took most of his knowledge to the grave — or more precisely, to the pyre. I have heard this scenario is playing out all over India. He tried to pass his calling on to his son, but for a variety of reasons, the transmission was incomplete. Few people in modern India, with its burgeoning middle class and growing

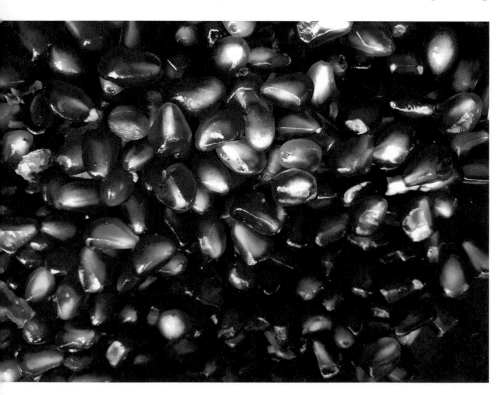

consumer sensibilities, want to make the kind of lifelong commitment required to reach Chandukutty's level — or even a fraction of it. Fewer still are starting their training as he had, as toddlers. And as with the violin, even committed students who start later never catch up.

———————

Even though I have little constant pain in my mouth two weeks in, I do have frequent episodes of shooting pain. If I cough, sneeze or — as I seem to be doing a lot — hiccup, I get a knife-stab of pain, but it passes as quickly as it arrives. I'm getting intermittent mouth dryness, but I seem to be digesting my meals without any difficulty.

Still, I lower the dose of herbs, matcha, and mushrooms, but combine them with the same amount of ghee. The resulting slurry coats my teeth, tongue, cheeks and, presumably, much of my soft palate. I let it linger in my mouth for as long as possible, tasting the complex mixture, which is nowhere near as bad as some I've had in both Ayurveda and TCM. My original motivation was the systemic effects of the herbs. Now, as with the oil pulling, I am thinking the local effects of the slurry on the mouth and throat might be even more important. Ayurveda would predict that much of the mixture would be absorbed directly into oral tissues.

———————

A dental resident at the hospital is repairing a cavity on an upper molar near the back of my mouth. He drills longer than I've ever experienced. Again and again, he pauses, then leans in for more. The procedure feels like it's taking much longer than it should.

I've known about the cavity for more than a month, but the hospital's dental clinic had no openings until two weeks into my RT. My doctors wanted me to use this clinic, rather than Tony and Madelyn's dentist, due to its experience working with oral cancer patients. It felt like a mistake to me to undergo a procedure when the tissues are under assault from chemoradiation, but the dental clinic insisted it wouldn't be a problem, and Dr. Clark agreed.

I can tell the resident is nervous. I imagine there is cold sweat beneath his purple latex gloves. As a medical intern, I had to do a few procedures that I didn't feel prepared for — and I remember how intimidated I felt. Just as I suspect the dentist is doing now, I tried to fake it.

My mouth has been feeling dry for the last several days, but it's parched now because I have to keep it open the entire time he works. As he drills, my skull vibrates like a jackhammer, far beyond anything I've experienced in a dental chair. Nor have I ever noticed any such procedure being especially loud. This is excruciating. It is a physical and aural assault.

That night my symptoms are decidedly worse. My voice sounds weak and froggy. My chin looks redder than usual, as does my neck. My face isn't puffy, but it's moving in that direction. For the last couple of days, I've been unable to eat or drink anything hotter than luke warm. I'm still making some saliva, but now I've got pain when I swallow.

The next day I start a prescription for a "stomatitis cocktail" to deal with the inflammation in my mouth. The banana-flavored syrup contains Decadron, in this instance used to reduce swelling and inflammation. It's also got viscous lidocaine (a topical anesthetic) and nystatin (an antifungal agent used as preventive medicine against thrush). The cocktail does provide some pain relief when I swish it around my mouth right before I eat. I do not, however, swallow it as my doctors suggested. I don't want to absorb any more Decadron into my system than is absolutely necessary. After a few minutes of swirling it around, I spit it out.

My discomfort is no doubt primarily from the chemoradiation, but I believe I got walloped harder because I didn't follow my intuition and instead listened to my doctors' and dentists' reassurances. Confirming my hunch, two days after the dental procedure the pain and dryness lessened, even though I'd received more RT each of those days, which should have increased those symptoms.

Had it turned out to be a routine procedure, I'm sure I would have done as well as was promised. So partly, it was just bad luck. But either way, I know I would have endured the procedure better if it had been done before my mouth was already a mess.

———————————

In the midst of my treatment for cancer, I'm continuing to work to rehabilitate my leg. It's part of the whole that I'm trying to make better. When I work with people in yoga therapy, my approach is usually directed at several areas simultaneously. Cancer is clearly the main thing I'm dealing with right now, but it's not the only thing.

As I practiced yoga the other day, my body sent me a signal. I tried a pose I hadn't done for a while. Kneeling on all fours, I lifted my left arm in front of me, and my right leg behind me, in a cross-crawl motion. I came down and switched sides. To my surprise, each time I lifted one arm and the opposite leg, I had difficulty keeping my pelvis from tipping to the side. I hadn't realized it, but presumably due to my quadriceps injury, my core muscles, which stabilize the torso, must have weakened. Luckily in yoga, the same exercise that reveals a weakness can also be its medicine. I started practicing the pose every day.

Today, out for a walk in the nature preserve near the house, crossing a gently upsloping hill, I spontaneously break into a jog. I continue for a hundred yards, and do this a couple of times, without problems. It's the first time I've run in more than six months. The long grass cushions each step. I am thrilled.

During my second week of treatments, a rash appears on my neck and face. There are little red bumps, inflamed skin and early on it started to scab. It's getting worse every day. There is not much pain, but it is unsightly. I mentioned the rash to Dr. Clark at our weekly appointment.

"Did you notice that it isn't over the parotids?"

He hadn't told me he was planning to shield these vital salivary glands, as I'd requested, and it's only in this moment that I realize he's done it.

Early on in my radiation treatment, when my pain is mild, Dr. Clark hands me a prescription for a liquid form of oxycodone, which surprised me, given all the negative publicity about opioids. He went straight for narcotics. I'd been expecting an approach more like, "Try a nonsteroidal drug like ibuprofen, and if that doesn't work, let us know."

He knows something that I do not about what lies ahead. From my doctoring days, I know that opioids can be very effective for acute pain. With the risk of addiction removed from the equation, as I feel certain it is, it seems like a good choice.

Dr. Clark lifts a handheld light and examines my mouth. After three weeks of treatment, he sees no trace of the tonsil. The tumor seems to be what he calls "radiosensitive," good news. The nodes, he says, are getting softer and smaller.

We continue our conversation about how much radiation I should get. He doesn't feel comfortable going to less than 60 Gray on the left tonsil, and favors 66 on the right neck metastases. I am still thinking 56 to both, but figure I'll see how I feel as we get closer to that dose.

At home, though, I can no longer see my tonsillar area well as it's too painful to open my mouth wide. My tongue feels tethered in my mouth, and it hurts to stick it out at all beyond the lips. This is the day I give up the hot tub. Heat, Ayurveda says, can promote inflammation, which I've got, and it's getting worse.

When I look in the mirror, though, I notice that the contour of the right side of my neck, which a few weeks ago a discerning eye could see wasn't normal due to swollen lymph nodes, now looks fine.

———————

I've now completed four rounds of chemo and 18 days of RT, for a total of 36 Gray. More than halfway through my treatments, my voice is stronger but it's still froggy ever since the dental fiasco. My lips are severely swollen, like a silicone injection gone wrong, cracked and scabbed over, especially first thing in the morning. My face from the cheeks down is thick and smooth, and I'm sporting a new jowly look. My neck is also puffy, with even less beard pushing through than the week before.

I have almost no saliva. I need to drink water throughout the day, and at night as well to keep my tissues moist. Even still, when I wake up my throat is so swollen that I can barely swallow water. So I start my day with a swig of the numbing suspension, swirl it around for five minutes, and spit it out. For a few minutes after that, swallowing is easier.

Two days ago, I began ibuprofen, 600 milligrams three times per day, which Dr. Clark recommended for the swelling. I was not expecting much from it. I'd prescribed that very dose hundreds of times in my medical career, mostly for musculoskeletal complaints like shoulder tendinitis, and never felt it did that much. But I think it's starting to help.

Within days my lips are less swollen, though I still have areas of dried purple blood, especially on the bottom lip. The skin on my neck, front and back, is more inflamed and scabbed over — red bumps pepper my chin and cheeks. The radiation dermatitis extends in a line beneath my collar bones in front and three inches or so beneath the shoulder line in back.

The worst spots are over the lymph nodes on both sides of my neck, especially the lower portion on the right side, near the collar bone. That's the location of the lowest and the most ominous of the cancerous nodes, as far as my prognosis goes.

The radiation also damages hair follicles. I've already lost the hair at the back of my head from the bottoms of my ears down. It looks like a bad bowl haircut. My beard is disappearing on my neck, and thinning on my face. When my skin started to get bad last week, I mentioned to Dr. Clark that I thought I'd grow my beard in. He didn't say anything, but I'm imagining he knew that wasn't likely.

Nothing I can do about the hair. But I start applying various salves — aloe vera gel, arnica, and calendula, which is made from marigolds — to see if I can soothe the rash on my skin. None of them are of much help. Then I try the Vicco turmeric cream I brought from India, which seems magical. Over the next few days, the skin on my neck starts to improve. This is not supposed to happen. With the ongoing assault from the RT, which is said to be cumulative, the rash should be getting worse, but just the opposite is occurring.

The cream comes in a sandalwood oil base, which is said to help deliver the turmeric more deeply into tissues. Both traditional Ayurvedic treatments, turmeric and sandalwood oil have pitta-calming, anti-inflammatory properties. I love the dry aromatic smell of sandalwood, though this product reminds me a bit of the flowery perfumes my great Aunt May used to wear. She was my favorite.

Over the course of the next week, I start laying on the pale yellow turmeric cream ever more thickly, and the rash drinks it in. It's as if the skin knows exactly what it needs. Within a minute of my troweling on the salve, the skin over the nodes toward the base of my neck shows through. So, I cake on another layer and that, too, is gone within minutes. Nearby, less-inflamed areas look as they had when I first applied the cream, having absorbed little. I end up reapplying the cream on the hot spots four or five times and start doing this several times a day.

"What are you doing to your neck?" the radiation therapy technician asks as I lie on the tomo platform. At first, I think she's detected some problem, but then I get it. She's amazed that despite the ongoing treatment, my skin has been steadily improving over the last week. She wants to try the turmeric cream on a skin condition of her own, which has nothing to do with RT. I spell the company's name for her and she writes it down.

I have used the same turmeric cream on precancerous spots on my face, known as actinic keratoses. Dermatologists typically freeze those off in the office. Just a few days of cream on the affected area of my cheek, though, and the redness disappeared and became smooth to the touch. It started to come back a year or two later, and I treated it again, and have had no recurrence in the several years since.

Chandukutty Vaidyar also made turmeric preparations, which I tried years ago in Kerala. His are likely more effective than the commercial product I'm using. But there's a big problem with them that might be familiar to you if you've ever cooked with fresh turmeric root. It stains your skin, your clothing, and anything else it touches bright yellow. Vicco has figured out how to make a turmeric product that rinses off.

Unlike the radiation therapy tech, none of my doctors seems the least bit interested in the turmeric cream that's making such a difference with my radiation burn. Maybe to them my experience is just an anecdote — and therefore not worth investigating — but I feel that this is something that's completely safe that might help many of their patients. Instead they recommend — and give me free samples of — a petroleum-based skin cream manufactured by a pharmaceutical company.

I have no intention of using it, especially at a time when my ulcerated skin is more permeable than usual. Because the skin is such an effective vehicle for absorption, doctors use it to deliver hormones, nicotine, and nitroglycerine via patches. I follow the advice of Ayurveda, and never put anything on my skin that I couldn't eat.

———————

Now during RT, I'm doing less chanting and I've added a visualization — an elaboration of the chi gung visualization that my med school buddy Srijan gave me — I've added breath holding. I imagine, with each slow inhalation, that my left tonsil and the nodes of the right side of the neck are on fire. As I hold my breath the flames burn brighter. I exhale gray smoke until my lungs are empty of breath and hold again, as I see the tissue burnt to ash.

But due to increasing inflammation, now I embellish it further. I don't want to just burn up the cancerous tissue. I want the normal tissue in harm's way to be nourished and protected. With the next inhale I imagine cool water flowing in and, as I hold the breath, the water removes the ash. As I exhale, the darkened water pours out, revealing healthy pink tissue beneath. I hold my breath and that tissue gleams.

With the next inhalation, I imagine fire again, repeating the cycle.

The yoga pose that is proving most helpful to me is one that I've rarely seen taught, except in Iyengar yoga classes, and even there only sparingly. Although this pose is typically done on a yoga mat on the floor, I've been doing it on my bed, which is softer and warmer. It's a prone twist called Supported Bharadvajasana.

I lie on the left side of my hips on the bed, with my knees bent, and one leg stacked on top of the other. My abdomen and chest turn toward the left so they can rest flat on a bolster. My head turns back toward the right, in the direction the knees are pointing, and my left ear rests on the bolster. Once I'm fully in the pose, I let go of everything. My breath deepens, as I sink in.

This deep stretch is focused on the very tissues of my neck threatened by the chemoradiation. And because it is what's known as a restorative pose, no effort is required. In restoratives, props like blankets, blocks and bolsters hold you up. All you have to do is lie there to get the benefits. Since I can hold the pose for a long time, the tissues relax even more.

Lately, I've been tired, and most days unable to do much yoga. Some mornings, just standing and lifting my arms overhead feels like too much. But this pose I can do no matter how depleted I feel. I stay 20 minutes, and then repeat it on the other side. Yesterday, Madelyn caught me asleep in the pose. I might have been there 45 minutes. Normally, that never happens.

I have had to give up Legs up the Wall, my go-to restorative pose, because it causes phlegm to build up in my mouth. In this pose, my body is in the shape of the letter L: my torso is horizontal, and my legs are vertical, supported by the wall. If I stay more than a minute in this position, I start to cough. My mouth is so inflamed that coughing is excruciating. This last week, lying flat on my back for RT has been hard to bear.

———————

As I expected, Madelyn has been offered the job up north. This is fabulous news, and I'm thrilled for her. I doubt it's been easy for Tony and Madelyn to have me here, and I'm aware that this is going to make everything more challenging. On top of their busy jobs, they will have to organize the move. All of their possessions will need to be packed up, and the house prepared to sell.

I'll have to leave six weeks after finishing my treatments, a few weeks earlier than I otherwise might have. I'm going to try to be helpful in any way I can, or at least be underfoot as little as possible, as workers, potential buyers, and finally movers come and go.

———————

Just before my fourth chemo infusion, with the side effects mounting, I email my friend and colleague Claudia and ask if she might advise me. She's trained in both Ayurveda and TCM, and is a smart clinician. We set up an online video chat. She ends up recommending two Chinese herbal medicines that I'm able to find online. Both are designed, as TCM sees it, to lessen the fire, which makes perfect sense considering the inflammation from the RT. She also recommends a salve for the radiation dermatitis.

Martha, my acupuncturist here, tells me she has been using needles and moxibustion to increase the water element with her treatments, which would metaphorically douse the fire. But she decides on each day's treatments only after she methodically takes my pulse, and she judges the success of each by assessing the pulse again after she's finished.

———

One of the biggest changes that came from yoga, which is helping me get through chemoradiation, is nasal breathing. With a few exceptions, almost all yoga practices are done while breathing through the nose. Before I started my yoga practice, I had been primarily a mouth breather, even when I slept. That dries the mouth and throat, which would have exacerbated the dryness I'm suffering now. Nasal breathing slows the respiratory rate, which in turn calms the nervous system. When the nervous system is relaxed, the mind tends to let go. All of that is helping.

All my life, I breathed through my mouth because it was easier. I had a deviated septem and bad hay fever due to ragweed, and not far away from where I lived in Milwaukee was the nation's ragweed epicenter, Kettle

Moraine State Forest. I never made a conscious effort to end mouth breathing. I just learned to breathe in a better way on my yoga mat, and practiced it enough that it took over, even during sleep. And then, one year in Kerala, Chandukutty gave me a spicy mixture of Indian culinary herbs that I was to put into raw local honey once I got home. I took one spoonful of the mixture every morning. It worked like magic. After using it a few years, I was able to stop it for a few years with no return of symptoms, until I need it again.

After the latest round of chemo — my fifth and likely second-to-last infusion — almost everything tasted bizarre. More foods are becoming impossible. I end the fast after my Thursday morning RT session with a beautiful fresh-pressed juice of organic vegetables and fruit. I take a sip and have to spit the green liquid into the sink because it burns my mouth so painfully. The next day I try a smoothie, which burns my mouth, too, but nothing like the juice. If any liquid lingers in the mouth, it hurts, so I start washing my mouth with a sip of water after each slug of smoothie, and I'm able to get it down.

I try poached eggs with toast. Even though I make the toast soggy with ghee, the texture is abrasive. I can't eat it. I try again without the toast, adding only ghee and salt. The salt burns some, but I'm happy that I've got something that still tastes normal.

Lying in the tomo machine, halfway into today's session, I noticed the faint aroma — meat on a grill. *It's the smell of my tongue cooking from the radiation.* I remember my shock as a third-year medical student when I first scrubbed in for surgeries. The electro-cautery device, the Bovie, which surgeons use to staunch bleeding capillaries, created a smell distressingly similar to the aroma of a barbecue. I'm not saying it was cause and effect, but by my fourth year of med school, I had become a vegetarian. Dr. Clark doesn't think it's possible that I was actually smelling my tongue, but I am not so sure.

———————

A guitar-playing dentist, who I met last summer at a chi gung workshop, emails me with a suggestion. Some of his patients with mouth pain have benefitted from what he calls "magic mouthwash." It a prescription medication that consists of a combination of equal parts milk of magnesia, a local anesthetic, and a liquid version of the antihistamine Benadryl.

He sends me a bottle in the mail, and it lives up to its billing. I swish it around my mouth for several minutes and find it more effective at relieving pain than the stomatitis cocktail Dr. Clark prescribed. I start alternating the two several times each day.

Initially, Dr. Clark expresses concern that the Benadryl will be too drying to my mucous membranes. Perhaps because I spit it out instead of swallowing it, though, I never experience that, which I tell him. When the bottle is running out, he is happy to renew the prescription.

———————

Last week Madelyn cooked an Indian curry, peas, and a little spinach with paneer cheese. I couldn't eat the peas but the paneer worked and, to my amazement, so did the spinach. It had been part of a failed smoothie attempt and I hadn't tried it separately since. So, today she cooks up a big batch of spinach and paneer curry for dinner, but the spinach burns my mouth and I can't eat it. This is frustrating for both of us. She has been trying so hard to help me, but the target seems to be moving ever further away.

Lying in the tomo machine, I feel a cough coming on, which I try to suppress. I don't want move an inch during the blast of radiation. If that happens, the ionizing rays would go where they are not intended, potentially damaging normal tissue and not the cancer. Somehow, I make it through, but it is torturous.

As soon as they unfasten the bolts that fix my head to the ramp, I tell the technicians I need a new mask. The swelling of my face has progressed so much that the mask squishes my face. It feels oppressive. Fluid collects in my throat as I lie flat — and I worry that I could suffocate. In response to my complaints, they get out a heat gun and subtly alter the shape of the mask.

The next day's session proceeds without problems.

As I walk to the door at the end of our weekly meeting, Dr. Clark places his hand on my shoulder and says, "Okay, brother." Every week when I see him, he uses some variation on this fraternal salutation. I feel understood and taken care of in those moments. It moves me.

Dr. Clark and his nurse Amy, another pitta kapha, are busy — everyone in health care is, but I never get the feeling that they don't have time to talk if it's important. When I was trying to decide on my treatments, I emailed him with questions. He suggested I call him at the clinic. He spent 40 minutes on the phone with me. No bill. Just being a great doctor.

Although it may not be recognized by insurance companies or evidence-based studies, this is part of what makes him effective: he is a doctor and a healer. His toolbox is strictly reductionist but he wields it in a compassionate and reassuring manner that likely improves his patients' well-being, and I'd guess, even their outcomes. With his kindness, and grounded compassion, he reduces his patients' fears, calms their autonomic nervous systems, and quiets their minds. All of that could improve immune function and cut inflammation — both of which are exactly what I need right now.

I managed to miss auricular acupuncture for the second week in a row. That treatment is painful. Several spots on both ears are exquisitely sensitive when Martha pierces the skin with the needles. The session is also held in the early evening, and that's a time I'd rather be home.

I'm wondering, though, whether the real problem could be the vibe. The ambiance of the windowless conference room in the city's health department, where the treatments are given, is less than ideal. The room has fluorescent lights (thankfully, switched off when we're there), mounds of stackable chairs, synthetic carpet and stale air. That carpet I would discover was not very clean either. Rather than sit in one of the chairs for the hour as most of the other patients do, I lie on the floor in a restorative yoga pose.

None of that was consciously behind my missing the appointments. I just got distracted and forgot — but I wonder if part of me didn't want to go. There is evidence that surgery patients who recuperate in a hospital room with a window that looks out on tree-lined courtyard heal more quickly, and get discharged sooner, than their compatriots who are warehoused in typical hospital rooms. I wasn't thinking about any of that, but some deeper source of knowing may have figured it out. The conference room just didn't feel as healing as Martha's lovely office, or the community clinic where I saw her, with its tasteful Asian decor.

———————

My mouth is sorer than ever. I'm now off the slurry of herbs that I'd been taking, though I'm still doing the oil pulling. I haven't tried juice again, but I am still hoping that smoothies will work. Yesterday, I added organic yogurt and cream-top milk back into my diet. As my dietary options dwindled, it felt like time to revisit the decision to cut dairy. I need to eat something to try to avoid losing too much more weight. I am committed to not getting a feeding tube — which the doctors have mentioned as a

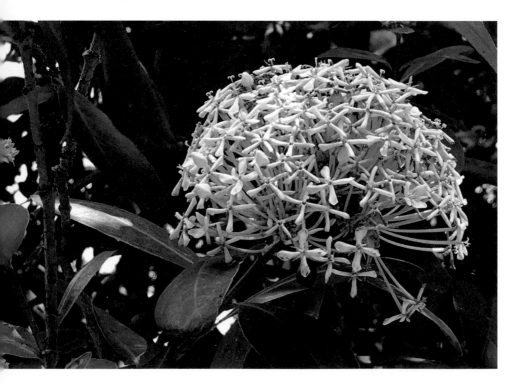

possibility — and finding something else I can eat could help me avoid that fate.

Linda, my artist friend from Burlington, Vermont, emails with a suggestion: custard. Her mom made it for her when she had a sore throat as a girl and was unable to eat. There would be eggs for protein, she says, and I could make it sweet or not. Madelyn gets out a classic cookbook from her prodigious collection, and cooks a liquid-y crème anglaise with just enough sugar to set the eggs. It goes down like silk. No pain at all.

She starts making large batches of it, and leaving it in the fridge. I am excited about this dietary discovery. The last time I tried poached eggs they still tasted normal, but I am getting sick of them.

I start thinking I should move to Burlington when I'm done here. Somehow, it just feels right. I try to find a place to live there, but the trusty Craigslist ad that's brought me three great apartments in the past — "Doctor/Author/ Yogi seeks..." — hasn't yielded much. Linda reposts it on an online community forum, and much better possibilities come in, including two on a street I remember well. It's a sleepy block in an artsy neighborhood, where Linda lived before and after she met my college buddy Mark. I'd visited them there many times, starting back when I was a medical resident.

She and Mark kept the place after they moved out, and have been renting it ever since. But when I started thinking of moving back to Vermont, where I'd spent so much time as a kid, I didn't even ask — it's a great place, and the tenants tend to stick around.

The next morning Linda texts: "Stop the presses. Our tenants just gave notice for May 1!" This is exactly when

I had hoped to move there, about six weeks after I finish treatment. This feels like a sign. I'm supposed to return to Vermont and the universe is confirming it. I don't remember much about the apartment itself, except that I liked it and it's where their older boy Cody was home-birthed.

I text her back: "I'll take it!"

Now that I've finished five rounds of chemo and 46 Gray of RT, my face looks much less swollen, as do my lips, though I've still got some scabs on my lower lips. That's from the ibuprofen, which is a happy surprise. My pain and swallowing problems have gotten worse, though. I am drinking all my food: poached eggs that I bowdlerize with a utensil from Madelyn's kitchen, and the crème anglaise. Smoothies are no longer possible.

The rapid response of the tonsil, no longer visible at three weeks, makes me decide it would be okay to stop at 60 Gray there. Dr. Clark thought my idea of 56 Gray was not enough. I'm more concerned about the metastatic nodes, which due to ongoing mutation tend to act more aggressively than primary tumors. I decide to go with Dr. Clark's suggestion of 66 Gray on that side of the neck, the lower end of current treatment recommendations. This would mean only one more infusion of chemo and ten more days of RT.

On the other side of my neck, halfway up, there's also one node of concern. It's enlarged but it looked normal on the ultrasound and the MRI, and it didn't light up on the PET scan. The left side is the usual location for metastases from a left tonsillar cancer, though, so Dr. Clark thinks we should treat that node, too. He suggests we go to 60 Gray there and 50 on the rest of that side, which I accept. Since Dr. Clark has allowed me to personalize the regimen, I am guessing that I'm the only one who has ever had this exact combination of doses.

I am happy with this plan. When I say this to Dr. Clark, he responds that it's a good compromise — though from his tone, I surmise he would have been happier if I'd gone to 70 Gray all around.

———————

It's hard to maintain weight. My appetite is lousy. I'm still fasting. The only things I can eat, I have to drink. I'm already too skinny. But I want to continue the fasting because I have no nausea from the chemo. Even if fasting isn't increasing the effectiveness of the chemoradiation, as I hope it is, it would be worth it to me just for its effect on nausea. Also notable is that I have no evidence of "chemobrain," the foggy cognition that cancer patients frequently report. Not for one second during this treatment have I felt anything other than mentally normal, and it wouldn't surprise me if fasting is helping there, too.

Fasting just feels right. The recommended foods do not. Throughout the treatment, my doctors have encouraged me to eat ice cream, pastries, and processed junk food — anything that's calorie dense to limit the inevitable loss of weight. As I wait to be called in for my chemotherapy and radiation treatments, hospital volunteers circulate through the waiting area with a cart offering free beverages like lemonade and punch — most loaded with sugar. The liquid nutrition supplements the doctors and nutritionists recommend, which are poured into the feeding tubes of the patients who opt for them, are, from my perspective, little better than junk food: sugar-laden, low prana, vitamin-fortified crap. There seems to be little consideration of how well any of these sugary offerings build healthy bodies. They are called empty calories for a reason.

On a couple of occasions, based on my blood test results, Dr. Shanahan wanted me to come in to get intravenous fluids. She writes in an email, using the lingo physicians use with each another, that she thinks I'm "dry." But the clinic is on the other side of town, and I don't feel like the hassle. Plus, I'm convinced that if I put my mind to it, I can drink enough fluid to rehydrate myself.

I can just feel in my bones that the more I continue to use my swallowing muscles throughout the treatment, the less likely I'll have problems getting food down once the treatment is finished. Swallowing difficulty is a common side effect, which sometimes persists for years.

That's also why I was so determined not to have a feeding tube surgically implanted in my stomach. A small percentage of people who get the tubes become dependent on them, for life — because their bodies forget how to swallow. I think it's important to have to use my mouth and throat, even though it hurts to chew and swallow. In yoga, we learn to endure short-term discomfort — like getting up to practice when we'd rather linger in bed — to get benefits later. This feels like an example of that.

I'm scheduled for my last RT session of the week, the treatment that would bring the total radiation dose so far to 54 Gray, but I feel like I've reached my limit. Yesterday the pain had gotten bad enough that I began to take the narcotics that Dr. Clark had prescribed in the second week.

One of the radiation techs calls. The tomo machine has gone down. They don't know if it will be repaired in time for my session today. A couple of hours later, I learn that it will not be. This means I will get a 96-hour reprieve between yesterday's treatment and Monday's. It feels like a gift.

———————

I am just learning in my research about a potentially debilitating long-term side effect of chemoradiation: fibrosis. This is stiffening in any of the tissues of the neck including the esophagus, which transports food to the stomach, and it may appear years later. Fibrosis can cause pain, swallowing difficulties and it sounds debilitating. I ask Dr. Clark about what I might do to prevent it. His response shocks me: "You know more about that than I do."

When I think about it later, his assertion — likely true — reflects a sad state of affairs. Somehow our medical education system has determined that it's not important for someone like Dr. Clark, a caring clinician, to be educated about non-drug options that might prevent a terrible side effect of the treatments he employs every day. Of course, if there were a drug that could decrease the risk, Dr. Clark would have known all about it.

But because all the treatments that are likely to work — like yoga, Ayurveda, and bodywork — have been relegated to the not-highly-regarded world of alternative medicine, they aren't on most physicians' radar. Patients never even learn there might have been something they could have done to prevent this awful aftereffect. And once fibrosis does set in, where holistic measures again might help, their clinicians may tell them that there are no treatments for it.

Even before getting radiated, my neck wasn't normal. The MRI revealed significant arthritic changes in the cervical spine, and stenosis — a bony narrowing of the canal that houses the spinal cord. Likely, both these are the result of childhood accidents. Although yoga has helped,

I can't turn my head all the way to the right. This poses problems when I'm driving and need to crane my neck to spot oncoming traffic from behind on that side.

Throughout my treatment, I have been doing yoga-inspired range-of-motion exercises for my neck, face, tongue and mouth — mindfully working to maintain freedom of movement. My flagging stamina limits how much I can do, but every day I manage some, including that restorative twist that stretches the neck.

Chanting is more preventive medicine. I chant for a variety of reasons, but one is the sound vibrations that resonate through the tissues of the head and neck. They've been healing in the past, and I think that they could be again. As I change the chants I recite and alter their pitch and volume, the effects vary, so I mix it up in order to stimulate different areas. I feel higher pitches vibrating in the nasal cavity, lower pitches in the neck.

Just before I chant, I do a practice called Bee Breath. With my lips closed I make a buzzing sound, which I can vary in pitch and volume as I do with chanting — directing the vibrations to different areas. With my mind alone — as yoga would predict — I can also change which tissues vibrate and bring focus on the areas threatened by the RT. Since the humming lengthens the exhalation, which is tied to the parasympathetic nervous system, it also tends to be relaxing. This has been my favorite yogic breathing exercise for years.

———————

When I started yoga, I was not into chanting. Perhaps it was the lingering effects of years of forced prayers in Latin at Masses that felt as cold and hard as the blond pews we sat on. Om, I liked, but not so much the droning verses of the *Yoga Sutras* that we recited in class.

Something changed after my first trip to India. Some of the chanting I heard there — with the warbling vocal inflections based on Indian musical scales — was gorgeous and haunting in a way the Sanskrit chanting I'd experienced in America was not.

At a yoga ashram near Bangalore, I learned to chant the mantra Om by intoning three sounds A, U and M. In some old books, that's how they write the word. A in Sanskrit is pronounced Ah, U rhymes with boo, and M is hummed at the lips.

At home, I'd chant the three letters separately and I noticed that I felt each sound in a different part of my body. When I said Ahhhhhhh, the resonance was strong in the belly, and I could feel it all the way down to the pelvic floor. Ooooooooo radiated out from the throat. Mmmmmm resonated all through the soft palate, mouth, and tongue.

I started putting them together: Ahhhhhhhhhh-ooooooooooooooo-mmmmmmmmmmmmm. And then it hit me: the ancient yogis didn't invent Om — they found it. It's built into the human body.

Yogis for millennia have aimed to raise pranic energy up the spine from the perineum to the crown of the head. When I chant A-U-M, I can feel the sound vibrations tracing that route. This is particularly true, I discovered, if you chant not three discrete sounds but rather open your throat fully for the A, gradually narrow it to form the U, then close your mouth to sound the M. Sliding from low to high, it's more like a trombone than a trumpet.

———————

The day of my sixth and final infusion of Cisplatin, my lab tests reveal that my immunosuppression has gotten worse — most noticeably the lymphocyte level has plummeted. Dr. Shanahan opts to reduce the dose of Cisplatin from the usual 40mg to 30mg. Even so, this means that I will have received a total of 230mg, a greater cumulative dose than many high-dose intermittent chemo patients manage to get. Once again, I feel no ill effects whatsoever as it's infused, although I know that by potentiating the RT, the chemo is contributing to all the side effects I'm experiencing, day in and day out.

My left nostril clogs every night with blood clots. It started with blowing blood-tinged mucus from my nose the second week of treatment. It felt to me like this was coming from the lower parts of the left side my nasal passages, which I figured was close enough to my cancerous tonsil to be irritated by the radiation.

But every morning I do a nasal wash with a neti pot — a little jug with a spout through which a saline solution flows into one nostril and out the other — and that seems to clear it up. Afterwards, I am able to breathe through that nostril all day. This is one ancient yogic treatment that has found its way into the mainstream. You can buy a neti pot at your local drugstore.

Three days before completing my cancer treatment, I take a selfie that I send out to my friends and family in my weekly email update. I'm wearing my maroon cap, still trying to stay warm, even in the house. My eyes are clear and I'm smiling brightly. Except over my sideburns, which haven't been affected much, I have only a few nubs where my beard used to grow in.

I am having significant pain, but the opioids I started a few days ago are helping. Even though the chemoradiation has been difficult, and my weight is way down, I look healthier in this photo than one taken the day before the chemoradiation commenced six weeks ago. My theory is that even though I had no obvious symptoms, I've had metastatic cancer growing for years, which was subtly undermining me. Now with the cancer in retreat, and maybe gone, even in the face of ongoing side effects, I'm better.

———————

To make up for my missed RT session, I am scheduled to get the final dose on a Monday. I tell Dr. Clark that this makes no sense to me. The treatments have a cumulative effect in damaging cancer cells. If there's a 72-hour delay between the second-to-last treatment on Friday and the final treatment, I say, it seems like I'd miss some of this benefit. Dr. Clark agrees. We decide to schedule two RT sessions on my final Thursday, then finish on Friday, March 17 St. Patrick's Day.

For most of my life, I've told people that I don't need to wear green on the holiday to be Irish — but this year the day feels a little more special. They say my symptoms will continue to worsen for 10–14 days post-treatment, so I know that tomorrow I'm likely to feel worse than today.

But emotionally, after that final RT session, I feel like I've passed a milestone. Tony and Madelyn quietly celebrate it with me at the dinner table, though mostly I just watch them eat. Things are going to get worse before they get better, but I feel like I've begun the journey back — and that makes me feel better right now.

———————

Eight days after finishing my treatments, I get up hungry and realize that I've finished off all the crème anglaise that Madelyn left for me. I remember that a nutritionist, who Dr. Clark's nurse Amy suggested, had given me a carton of an organic protein drink, made by a company called Orgain. Amy sent me to this nutritionist specifically because I'd told her that there was no way I would drink the ones most nutritionists suggest.

I hadn't tried the carton after the nutritionist gave it to me, though. Weeks before that, I had bought a tub of Orgain's protein powder and mixed some into home-made almond milk — but it burned my mouth. I assumed the pre-mixed version would be the same. But I am desperate, so I go down to my bedroom and find the package. It's got more sugar than is ideal, but it's organic and it's made from real food.

It goes down smoothly with minimal discomfort. I feel overjoyed. I am so sick of custard and poached eggs, the only foods I've been able to eat. My weight is down 20 pounds from before I started chemoradiation — I look the skinniest I've ever been. Later that day, I drive into town and buy a half dozen cartons, in a few different flavors. Vanilla goes down smoothly, though I need to drink water after each sip to clear any remnants from my mouth. Otherwise it burns. Strawberries & Cream is a bit worse, but it's doable. Unfortunately, Chocolate tastes good, but it burns my mouth, and will have to wait.

Over the next two days, I ramp up from the 500 calories per day that I estimate I've been consuming for weeks. Late in my treatment I was horrified to learn that the three large eggs I'd been having for dinner most nights amounted to only 210 calories, plus whatever I got from the ghee. Finally, I'm getting to consume something that is not made from eggs, even if it's just a protein drink in a box.

———————

My friends Andy and Vicki visited last week, which I really enjoyed. Andy is also a writer, we share a love for music, and we're both on the path of self discovery. He and I can talk for hours. Off and on since the '80s, we've played music and sung together. They'd been down south to visit his aging mother, and took this route back to Vermont in order to see me. Mark and Linda, in the area to watch their younger son play lacrosse, came the week before that. Even though at that time, 10 days post-treatment I was near the peak of my pain, we were able to walk in the nature preserve. My nephew Jonathan and his partner Nithya also visited, during a break from teaching in Ecuador, which was especially nice because it was the first time I got to spend significant time with her. Regular phone calls to Andy and Tomas, my best friend from medical school, were another emotional lifeline, though about four weeks into treatment I'd had to give them up — I noticed my mouth was dryer and the pain was significantly worse after talking. I can still feel the love of my friends but other than these in-person visits, our interactions are mostly limited to email.

———————

Around the table after dinner one night, Tony sits eight feet from me. He is saying something to Madelyn. His lips are moving, but I hear no sound. My hearing has been getting worse, but this floors me.

I've decided that I've got fluid in my Eustachian tubes, behind both eardrums. If I pull on an ear just right, though, my hearing will suddenly get better. A minute later it's as bad as before. That tissue was close enough to the radiation target to get a significant dose, and it must still be inflamed.

———————

The first real food I am able to eat a couple of weeks

into recovery is a few ounces of salmon, with no spice, that Madelyn poaches for me. It goes down smoothly.

Days later, Madelyn prepares a mountain of pesto for a going-away party for themselves that they will be hosting at the house. Soon she will be heading north for the new job, though Tony won't join her right away. I have my doubts about the pesto, but not only can I eat it, it also tastes normal! Neither of those is a given these days. I have ingested nothing interesting from a culinary standpoint for a couple of months — and to taste the fresh basil, garlic, pine nuts, and parmesan is beyond words. It feels like another significant step on the way back.

Although my hearing is still muffled, by concentrating on people's lips, I manage to have a number of nice conversations at the party. Over the years they've been here, Tony and Madelyn have built a solid community in their adopted hometown. I can feel how well-loved they are. It's also clear how popular anything Madelyn cooks is. Long before my early bedtime, the platter of pesto resembles a mountaintop mine after the coal has been extracted.

Almost exactly one month post-treatment, I receive an invitation to give the keynote address next March at the annual conference of a large yoga organization in the UK. I hatch a plan. What if I fly to India beforehand to spend the tail end of my first year after chemoradiation getting intensive Ayurvedic treatments? They could help me overcome any lingering aftereffects, and would be preventive medicine for the path ahead.

I call Krishna. He suggests three months of treatments, which would be by far the most I'd ever had. Since I'll be teaching in Britain afterwards, he suggests we plan an additional 21 days of rest at the end. Although they may not look intense, Ayurvedic treatments can be depleting in the short term. I'd learned that lesson the hard way when I stopped to teach at an ashram in the Bahamas on the way home from Kerala one year — and came down with a debilitating case of influenza.

I book the plane tickets. I have no idea what kind of shape I'll be in by November, when it will be time to leave. Still, the plan feels perfect, and the keynote offers one of those gifts that falls from the sky when you need it. Because I had just taken additional funds out of my retirement savings to finance my medical care, the speaking offer had another benefit. While in England, I could teach a couple of workshops in London. Plus, the sponsors would pay my airfare to the UK, and by routing my trip through London, I could fly to Calicut for half what it would have cost me otherwise.

———————

Near the end of my stay, Madelyn brings up an issue that has bothered them. Four years ago, Tony ruptured both of his quadriceps tendons when he misjudged a step. Madelyn reminds me that she phoned me at the time and asked me to fly out from California to take care of him during the week of his surgery — but I had said I couldn't do it. At first, I don't remember that conversation.

Now that I've suffered the same injury — and can imagine how much worse it would be to have two of them simultaneously — I feel awful. Even though it would have been inconvenient for me to come, I know I should have done it. Considering how generous they have been to me in the past few months, I feel even worse. She suggests I apologize to Tony, as it has been something that's been hard for him to get past. A couple of days later, when Madelyn is out shopping, I find Tony reading the paper sitting on their bed. He's still dressed in shorts and shoes from his morning run. I tell him how sorry I feel. He shrugs, shakes his head, and says it's okay.

Ten days before I'm due to head out for Vermont, all traces of the skin rash are gone. I've put on five of the 20 pounds I've lost. I am still in pain, taking the opioids as needed, and tired, but I'm able to get out for gentle walks in the nature preserve most days. Some food still tastes bizarre, which Dr. Clark's resident tells me might never return to normal. I can see subtle swelling in my face, but no one else seems to notice. Madelyn has commented several times on how much healthier I look. This is welcome news, because when I move to Burlington, I'd prefer not to have to explain to every person I meet what's going on. If asked about my hearing problem, I figure that I'll just say I have fluid in my ears.

Although I didn't learn about it until after completing my treatment, there is a hypothesis, called the metabolic theory of cancer, that would explain why fasting could weaken tumors. And why, conversely, the foods that I've been urged to eat — all those high-sugar products — might actually fuel malignant growth. First advanced by the Nobel Laureate Otto Warburg in the 1920s, the theory fell into obscurity after Watson and Crick discovered the structure of DNA in the 1950s. A new theory that cancer is the result of mutated genes — oncogenes — became the prevailing dogma. But Warburg's theory, which is now again gaining some currency, posits that the chief cause is that cancer cells have severely damaged mitochondria.

In normal tissues, the mitochondria, oblong organelles

inside cells, act as power plants, metabolizing oxygen and generating energy for cellular functions. But the deranged mitochondria in cancer cells can't do this. Instead of burning oxygen like normal tissues, cancer cells rely on fermenting sugar to generate energy, which isn't as efficient, and causes a massive build-up of cellular free radicals. Those "reactive oxygen species," as they are known medically, may be the cause of the ongoing mutation in cancer cells.

No one disputes that cancer cells consume massive quantities of sugar, on the order of ten times normal cells. In fact, the uptake of sugar is what cancer-staging PET scans measure. The patient is injected with a radioactive glucose solution and the malignant sugar-gobbling cells light up, as my tonsil and lymph nodes did. Cancer cells need all this glucose because of their imperative to grow and grow. It just makes sense to me that when there's less of the fuel they need, cancer cells are going to have a harder time.

Though Warburg's idea languished in obscurity for many decades, he insisted until the end that he would be vindicated. The primary modern-day proponent of the metabolic theory of cancer is Professor Thomas Seyfried of Boston College. He believes that mutations in DNA, which are viewed as the cause of cancer, are instead *the result* of damaged mitochondria and the high levels of free radicals that are generated inside the cells during sugar fermentation.

Viruses, including HPV, have been shown to target mitochondria and alter their metabolic pathways. Mitochondria have their own DNA, different from what's in the cell nucleus. Whether or not deranged oxygen metabolism is the cause of cancer, it is beyond doubt that cancer cells are voracious — and obligate — consumers of glucose. Unlike regular cells, they don't have a low-energy mode.

Ingenious experiments, including some by Dr. Seyfried, offer support for abnormal mitochondria as the root cause of cancer. Scientists implanted the nuclei of cancer cells containing mutated DNA into normal cell bodies, full of healthy mitochondria. The resulting hybrids acted like normal cells and did not generate tumors. But when they did the opposite — transferred the nuclei of normal cells into the bodies of cancer cells that were full of damaged mitochondria — the resulting hybrids did generate malignancies, despite the normal DNA.

Cancer cells have many more insulin receptors on their surface, facilitating their prodigious uptake of sugar. Fasting lowers blood sugar levels, insulin levels, and levels of what's known as IGF-1, an insulin growth factor that like insulin is thought to fuel cancer. Once you've used up the body's sugar reserves, stored in the liver as glycogen — usually within the first 24 hours of fasting — the body shifts to living off fats, taken from the body's reserves. The liver packages stored fats into molecules known as ketone bodies. The state in which there are high levels of ketones in the bloodstream is known as ketosis.

Normal tissues in the body — as well as brain cells, which I was taught in medical school prefer glucose as their fuel — are in fact more than happy to live on ketones. They can do it indefinitely without harm. This combination of stressing cancer cells by depriving them of the fuel they desperately need, while providing plenty of fuel for the healthy cells, may account for fasting's purported ability to boost the effectiveness of both chemotherapy and radiation *and* lessen their side effects. While the metabolic theory of cancer has not been proved, if it does turn out to have some validity, the high sugar foods that were recommended during my treatments — foods that would have fed the appetite of the cancer cells for more glucose — might have been terrible advice.

Meanwhile, doctors like Tony have legitimate concerns about fasting, worried that any additional weight loss could undermine the chance of recovery. Fair enough. Let's study that. But why not also study the idea — which seems dubious to me — that it's a good idea during cancer treatment to eat low-quality, and typically high-sugar, food as long as it's high in calories? Somehow in modern medicine, the potential dangers of the standard advice tend to go unquestioned. It's often only the counter theories for which proof is demanded.

The summer after my treatments are finished I figure out that without planning to, toward the end of chemoradiation I had been in ketosis for days on end. Consuming only eggs, ghee, and full-fat milk, I was eating a so-called ketogenic diet. Due to the potential benefits of ketosis in suppressing cancer, this high-fat, moderate protein, low-carb diet — now widely used for weight loss — is touted for patients with malignancies. Looking back, I am guessing that I was in ketosis from near the end of February till eight days after I finished treatments, when I started the Orgain shakes. That's 27 days straight.

In addition, over the course of six-and-a-half weeks of chemoradiation, I did six 63-hour water fasts. It takes a while to go into ketosis, so let's assume conservatively that it took me 24 hours of fasting to reach ketosis each time. That would be 234 hours, nine or 10 days, of additional time the tumors would have had their meal ticket revoked. Each chemo and at least two RT sessions per week would have come when I was in a state of ketosis.

Any cancer cells in my body would have been deprived of almost all nutrition for weeks, while they were being bathed in Cisplatin and blasted with radiation. The therapeutic benefits of chemoradiation are cumulative, and continue to gain in potency in the initial days after the treatments cease. Thus, their anti-cancer effects would likely have peaked during those final days of ketosis, the week after I completed my treatments. If Longo's research on fasting in mice turns out to apply to humans, this prolonged period of ketosis would have increased the potency of the chemoradiation and with it, perhaps, my chance at a cure.

———————

My last day in town, I have an appointment with Dr. Morrison, the ENT surgeon. The first time we met, he urged me to have radical neck surgery. I haven't seen him since, but he learned from Dr. Clark that I'd decided against the operation. My car is already packed, and is parked in the clinic lot, ready to go.

Once again, I wait in a treatment room. The colorfully-tattooed nurse practitioner who works with Dr. Morrison arrives, and she wants to spray a local anesthetic into my nostrils. The doctor's plan is to thread a fiber-optic scope into my nose and down the back of my throat, she says, to look at my tonsil. This is the first I've heard of it. I balk. My tissues have been so traumatized by the treatments, I'm not sure it's a good idea. Besides, if the doctor wants to do a procedure, he should talk to me about it first.

Dr. Morrison seems irritated when he enters the room. I ask him a few questions, which he answers, and I agree to the procedure. I am perfectly willing to disappoint, or even piss off, my doctors, if that's what it takes to make sure I get only the care I need — and not an ounce more.

The exam goes well. He sees no trace of cancer. I ask him about my hearing loss. He agrees with my assessment that it's likely due to fluid in the ears.

"What do you suggest?" I ask.

"Ask people to speak up." While many patients might prefer some kind of medical intervention, this strikes me as sage advice.

When I'd told Dr. Morrison that pulling on my ears had helped my hearing, even if only temporarily, he had said that didn't make sense anatomically. I'd used this technique many times, and it had worked, but he doubted it was possible.

When I was little, my brother Ray told me that, given how fat their bodies are and how tiny their wings, "bumblebees theoretically can't fly." Which to me is evidence that we need a better theory.

That's the problem with modern medicine: Counterexamples, like my experience tugging on my ears, or healing my radiation rash with turmeric cream, are dismissed. They are nothing more than "anecdotal evidence" — evidence-based medicine's bête noire — and are never investigated. Opportunities to falsify prevailing theories — a major goal of the scientific method — or to expand the treatment armamentarium are systematically ignored. The door to new understanding is preemptively slammed shut.

That kind of thinking just won't work for me. I can't afford to dismiss any options that might end up saving my life or helping to restore its quality. I plan to keep the doors of perception wide open, as I continue to negotiate the tortuous journey back to health.

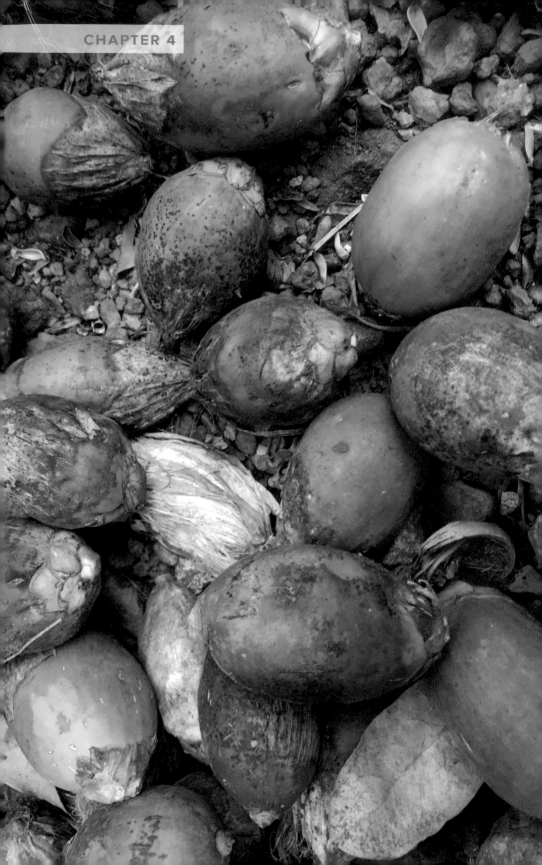

SKILL IN ACTION

Six weeks after my cancer treatment is finished, I move into half of a duplex in Burlington, Vermont. It's filled with light, and has hardwood floors and a big back yard. This feels like a very good place to be. Most of my stuff is still in storage in the Hudson River Valley, so I'll be driving a 26-foot moving truck down and back this weekend, and paying professional movers to load the truck for me — I still haven't returned to full strength.

My recovery continues to go well, though slowly. I don't have much pain. My appetite is not huge, but seems to be improving. I'm able to eat many solid foods, and have put on a few more pounds. Some items continue to burn my mouth, but I can't predict which ones. Last week I was able to eat spaghetti sauce, as well as salad with oil-and-vinegar dressing, which had previously caused problems. A slice of apple burned a bit, and a single red grape set my mouth on fire.

What affects me most is that I often can't understand what people say to me. The fluid in my ears continues to impair my hearing. My energy is up and down, but

I'm still doing yoga and walking. Gradual improvement seems to be the trend. I'm due to return to teaching in two weeks, with a five-day yoga-therapy workshop in Maine. I wouldn't have enough stamina to lead one now, but am hoping that by then I'll be able to pull it off.

―――――――――

After I settle into Burlington, I call Krishna to catch up. He'd read the group emails I sent out to close friends and family members during my treatment, but he hadn't responded to any of them. This is the first time we speak. I am thrilled to hear that Aiswarya is planning on applying to Ayurvedic medical college.

To gain admission, however, she will have to take an exam that is extremely competitive. She is an outstanding student but is at a disadvantage because the exam is in English, and her education has been at a Malayalam-language school in their rural community. Public schools in big cities and many private schools teach in English and have better-trained teachers.

Also taking this exam are the children of Indians residing in England, Singapore, the United States and other countries who would like to study medicine in India. Due to their English skills and superior educational opportunities, many of them have a huge advantage over a student like Aiswarya.

―――――――――

One thing that continues to concern me is the fibrosis I'd asked Dr. Clark about. He had no suggestions for preventing this feared aftereffect so I consult again with my friend, Dr. Claudia, who emails a suggestion: Try castor oil packs on my neck to make the tissues more supple. She says I might apply one once a week. Soon after I arrived in Burlington, she'd recommended daily castor oil massages, but I found the oil sticky and difficult to massage with — but the pack seems more doable.

I pour a half-dollar-sized puddle of the viscous oil with little smell into one palm, then rub my hands together to warm it. I massage the oil into both sides of my neck simultaneously, and for good measure over my thyroid gland and parotids.

Then I wrap a wool flannel cloth around my neck, tucking one end in to secure it. I cover that with a piece of plastic that I've cut from a store bag, again tucking one end above the upper edge. Finally, I take an old hand towel, fold it in half lengthwise and wrap it over the other two layers. I leave the pack on for 45 minutes. The flannel and its coverings keep the area warm, helping the oil penetrate into the tissues. They are safer than a hot pack, which Claudia says might damage the heat-sensitive thyroid tissue — already threatened from the chemoradiation.

The next day I have an idea. What if I put on the castor oil pack right before I sit to do my yogic chanting, breathing, and meditation? They usually take an hour, which would give the oil plenty of time to soak in. I start doing this several times per week, and within days I can tell that it's helping make the tissue suppler.

And then I have another idea: An acupuncturist I worked with a few years ago advised regularly massaging all scars with oil to improve the flow of chi. When I finish rubbing castor oil into my neck before applying the pack, I use the excess on my hands to massage a couple old scars from injuries and the one from the surgery on my left knee.

Three months post-treatment, I fly south and stay

with Tony at the now mostly-emptied house. Tony hasn't moved yet, but Madelyn is already on the new job up north. I drive back to the medical center for another PET scan to evaluate my response to the treatment. Within a couple of hours, I'm meeting with Dr. Clark.

Dr. Clark says that the areas that lit up on my initial test seven months ago, indicating cancer, have returned to normal. He examines me carefully and finds no evidence of cancer in my mouth or of any abnormal lymph nodes. I have had what they call a "complete clinical response."

Although this is the news I've been hoping for, Dr. Clark says that there's a five to 10 percent chance the cancer will recur in the first three years. This is worse than I'd thought. My recollection was that they'd told me I'd have a 90-95 percent chance of being cured before I started treatment, but I realize they must have said those were my odds of a complete clinical response. I can't believe I'd made that mistake.

Next, I go to see my oncologist, Dr. Shanahan. During our appointment, she asks me how I've been doing in the three months since finishing treatments. From her responses to my description, I glean that I have better function and fewer symptoms than most patients in my situation.

"You just sailed through your treatments," she says, smiling broadly.

I hadn't planned on revealing it all, but find myself asking, "Would you like to know why?"

Sure, she says.

"I fasted. I drank nothing but warm water for almost two days before each chemo session. That's why I didn't have any nausea and vomiting." I tell her about the case studies of patients with various cancers who'd tried different fasting regimens that I'd read in one of the oncology journals. I ask if she's heard about this. She has not, but she wants to know what else I had done.

Her interest surprises me, so I go with the opening. I mention how we use the breath in yoga to manipulate the autonomic nervous system (ANS) — how the inhalation stimulates the sympathetic response (SNS), while exhalation increases the parasympathetic tone (PNS). We use this ability to modulate and achieve balance in the ANS to affect every internal organ and various systems in the body. My training in medicine allows me to talk to Dr.

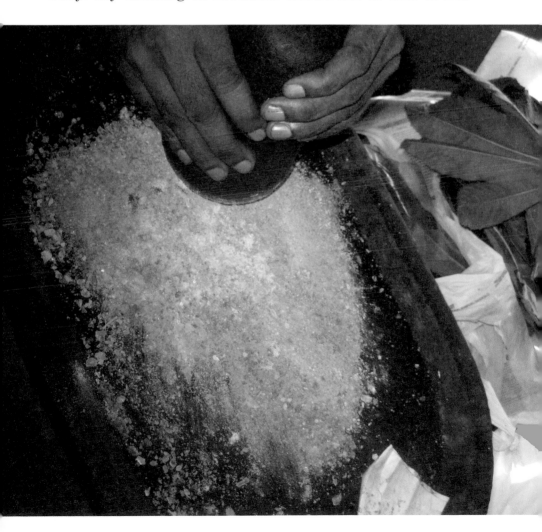

Shanahan in language that will sound familiar to her, and to provide credible scientific explanations of the mechanisms that are responsible for many of yoga's effects.

Dr. Shanahan seems fascinated. She tells me that she once took a mindfulness meditation course, which I find encouraging — and surprising. She had seemed so opposed to the gentle herbs and other treatments I had planned. I had assumed that she wouldn't be interested in mind-body approaches.

All told, she lingers an extra half an hour to talk about the modalities I'd used — a long time in the schedule of a busy doctor. I realize that she is more open-minded than I'd thought. The problem is that she was trained in a system that does not value — and often condemns on the basis of little real knowledge — many of the holistic methods that made such a huge difference in my getting through the treatment she so expertly and compassionately delivered.

––––––––––

At my first meeting with the ENT surgeon, Dr. Morrison, he had said that the likelihood that I would have a complete clinical response was excellent. "What happens in five to ten years, nobody knows." I have been reading that with this cancer, recurrences can happen years later and sometimes pop up in unusual locations like the kidneys, muscles, and skin.

Toward the end of the summer after my cancer treatment, the first study I've seen that evaluates the five- and ten-year survival of HPV oral cancers is released in a Canadian medical journal. I read it with great anticipation, and am crestfallen by the time I get to the end. Piecing together data from numerous institutions, the authors concluded that about 50 percent of patients were alive five years after diagnosis. At 10 years, the number dropped to 18 percent. This sounds a lot worse than what my doctors down south had indicated.

I am also aware that I had three "negative prognostic factors." My nodes were on the opposite side of my body from my primary tumor, one was down near the collar bone (a Level 4 node), and the MRI suggested the cancer may have broken through the capsule surrounding one or two of the lymph nodes. Weighing all of that, I figure it's highly likely that I would be in the 82 percent dead within 10 years group. It seems probable — even though my recent physical exam and PET scan were normal — that I have hidden micro-metastases.

I send the study to Tomas, my medical school buddy. He and I met at the picnic for incoming freshman, became anatomy lab partners, and lived on the same block for most of med school. We've been fast friends ever since. He reads the study carefully, and points out various ways in which the results may not apply to my case. I don't feel that reassured.

I email Dr. Clark, asking him if the study's findings comport with what he's seen in his own practice. He writes back to say that "the Canadian data is concerning," but does not say if the results match the experience of the patients he's treated. I find that concerning.

———————

The solar eclipse is coming. I've been taught in India that observing eclipses can weaken you. Yogis are advised to stay home and meditate during them, and normally that's what I try to do. But this time I figure that if I might not be around for the next full solar eclipse here, seven years hence, I'm going to watch this one. I decide to attend the event at the public library.

Hundreds of people are gathered on the lawn out front. The library supplies cardboard solar viewing glasses, but on this sunny day, demand far exceeds supply. I am fortunate to get a pair, sharing them with others throughout the event. A woman next to me holds a colander up to a sheet of cardboard, which creates gorgeous patterns of half-moon shadows. One of the people borrowing the glasses is a man I'd met at another library freebie, a Scandinavian black-bread-making workshop.

We were part of a group of three who mixed and kneaded the dough we got to take home and bake. He told me that he had early Alzheimer's disease, though it wasn't noticeable in our interactions. I was surprised at how open he was about his diagnosis. Normally I don't proselytize about yoga, but I told him that there is evidence that the practice may slow cognitive decline. I suggested that if he's interested, he should start soon to solidify the habit patterns before his memory gets any worse.

Habits are important. Anything you say or do or even think repeatedly, you are more likely to say, do, or think again. That's because each behavior causes neurons to forge connections with one another. The more the behavior is repeated, the deeper those neural networks become. Neuroscientists have a saying: "Neurons that fire together, wire together." Even though scientists just figured this out in the last 20 years, it's consistent with the ancient yogic understanding of forging new habit patterns.

In the *Yoga Sutras*, the second century text, the author Patanjali gave a formula for success in yoga: steady and enthusiastic practice over a long period of time without interruption. This is also the perfect formula to take advantage of neuroplasticity to rewire the brain. As Swami Vivekananda, the first yogi to come to America in 1893, put it: "The only remedy for bad habits is counter-habits."

A yoga practice can be the new habit that deepens with repetition until it gets so strong that it can out-compete old habits.

The crowd thinning, I head home while the eclipse is still visible. Before the sun shines unobstructed, I'm on the cushion in my yoga room, meditating.

———————

After I read the Canadian study, I come to believe that I need to "up my game." If I want to beat the odds, I need to do even more to create an internal environment that will inhibit the growth of cancer. In all likelihood, my clean lifestyle and yoga practice had helped keep the tumor in check for a while, perhaps for many years, but they obviously had not been enough.

My first target: sugar. After I returned to eating after treatment, rail thin and wanting to build myself back up, I enjoyed some ice cream and other desserts for a couple of months. Now, though, I eliminate all added sugars, as well as simple carbohydrates like white rice and white flour, which are rapidly metabolized to sugar. I give away bags of organic figs and dates.

I even cut out dark chocolate. Before the cancer, I'd consumed it nearly every day for years. Instead, I start adding unsweetened, organic cacao to my milky chai tea. The fabulous milk from a local family farm makes it just sweet enough, and I come to love it.

I also resolve to eat higher-prana food. This is easy to do in Kerala, where every meal I'm served is freshly prepared. Following Ayurvedic principles, Krishna's wife Bindu does not reheat food or use a refrigerator to store leftovers. If humans don't eat it by the next meal, she'll feed it to the animals.

But here in Vermont, particularly now that I'm living

alone again, I tend to make batches of curry or spaghetti sauce. Sometimes I eat leftovers a couple of days later, which is a no-no in Ayurveda. This advice is not realistic for many people, I realize. It's a burden for me at times, too, but right now I want to get everything aligned in the direction of being cancer-free. I start cooking fresh every meal.

I inherited a back-yard vegetable garden, and have been eating gorgeous organic chard and kale. Typically, I'll start to cook my lunch, and then go out back and harvest whatever vegetables and fresh spices I'm using. For spices like cumin and coriander that I don't grow, rather than use powders that may have been sitting in jars for ages, I grind the seeds fresh. I do the same for the flax seeds I sprinkle on my steel-cut oatmeal in the morning.

I come across a study that found that women with breast cancer who fasted overnight had 36 percent fewer recurrences. The advantage was seen in women who ate nothing for at least 13 hours, compared to those whose overnight fasts were shorter. Women with the longer intervals were found to have lower levels of hemoglobin A1C, a marker of the average level of their blood sugar. Other studies have found overnight fasting is associated with lower levels of inflammation.

For thousands of years, Ayurveda has taught that you should eat nothing between dinner, which it advises be completed by about 6:00 p.m., and breakfast. I've been following this advice for years, but after reading the Canadian study, I become more vigilant about eating nothing, not even a morsel, in the hours after dinner.

Since I do a yoga practice first thing in the morning, I typically don't eat till after 9:00 a.m., meaning at least 15 hours of fasting per day. All my calories are consumed in a nine-hour window between breakfast and dinner. Some people try to narrow that window further, but this feels

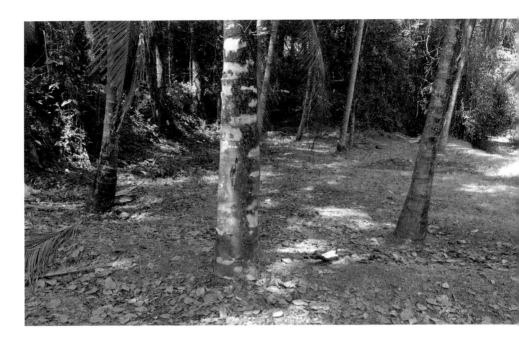

sufficient to me, especially since I'm still trying to put on the weight I lost during my cancer treatment.

Even so, I also decide to revisit the idea of water fasting. Despite the need to regain weight, the advantages of ketosis and autophagy from a brief fast might lower my risk of a recurrence. I figure that even if I lose a few pounds fasting, now that my appetite is normal and I have no mouth pain, I'll be able to put them back on quickly.

I decide to skip breakfast the next morning and see how I feel after that. I prepare a large thermos of warm lemon water and sip it all morning. At lunch I don't feel too hungry, so I keep going. I do the same at dinner. Meanwhile, I'm discovering that when you're not cooking, cleaning, and shopping for food, extra hours become available in your day.

With the additional time, I find myself studying fasting and the metabolic theory of cancer. I read an article by Dr. Seyfried, the theory's leading modern proponent, and watch a couple of his interviews online. He recommends a four- to seven-day fast every year as cancer prevention. I download a book on fasting and read it. I read another the next day. Two and even three days in, I'm still feeling good, with no hunger, though I find myself fantasizing about what I'll eat when I break the fast.

I do notice an increase in my heart rate, which I suspect is due to sympathetic nervous system activation from the lack of food. Probably for the same reason, I'm finding it harder to sleep. I'm averaging only six hours per night and, by the fourth day, I'm exhausted. On the positive side, I notice increased mental clarity — and have been unbelievably productive. I've checked off dozens of boxes on my to-do list for items that I'd been putting off for months.

On the fourth day, I decide I'll end the fast the next morning. All told, I go 111 hours without food. I lose two-and-a-half pounds, and put it back on within three days. Some of the weight reduction from fasting is due to water loss, they say, which may explain why I regain the weight so quickly. In retrospect, I feel like I probably went one day longer than I should have, but this feels like something I want to do again.

Six months after treatment, I follow up with an ENT doctor at a medical center in Burlington, Dr. Angelina Kuantai. She takes a detailed feel of my neck and puts on a latex glove to palpate the area around the tonsils. In addition, she scopes my throat through my nose, and thinks everything looks great. I'm impressed with how thorough her exam is.

My blood count has edged up to 35 from 33 at three months out, but is still 15 percent lower than normal. I still have some fatigue, most noticeable after I exercise. That's probably in part due to the anemia. My heart rate goes up very quickly, so I tell the doctor I've backed off on the aerobic exercise I'd been doing. I have no problems at all with writing and teaching and my usual daily activities.

I produce some phlegm every morning, so there's probably still inflammation in my mouth. I don't tolerate spicy food either. My sense of taste, though, has returned to normal — no foods taste "wrong" anymore. I'm thrilled this unpleasant side effect of chemoradiation, which took a lot of the pleasure out of eating, is gone. I was told it might never resolve.

One concern is that my thyroid hormone levels are barely normal, and the thyroid-stimulating hormone (TSH) is now elevated — I suspect I'm on the road to losing my thyroid. This is an aftereffect of the chemoradiation that I've been worried about. When the thyroid is starting to fail, the body makes more TSH to goose the gland to produce more hormones. I've read that the condition I've got, known medically as "subclinical hypothyroidism," is typically a stepping-stone to full-blown hypothyroidism. The latter generally requires life-long thyroid medication. I email Dr. Clark and asked him how much radiation the gland likely got. He answers 50 to 52 Gray — the amount in half-a-million chest X-rays. My research suggests that's more than enough to kill the thyroid.

But if losing my thyroid is the price of survival, it's a price I'm willing to pay.

———————

One sunny afternoon in the spring of 2014, my fiancée and I were lying in bed in my Oakland, California apartment. Her hand brushed my neck and then came to a stop. "What's this?" she asked.

I put my hand on the right side where she had indicated, just beneath the jaw bone. I felt an enlarged lymph node. It was firm, but not rock-hard or tender to the touch, and I could move it around with my fingers. I knew it was potentially worrisome — I'd felt many such nodes in my years of practicing medicine.

My first thought was lymphoma, though I didn't mention it to her. The cancerous disease of the lymphatic system can cause painless swollen lymph nodes like the one I had. At that time, though, I had just returned from a couple of months in Kerala, living around cows, goats, and chickens. I wondered whether I might have been exposed to some funky virus or bacteria that my body had reacted to. Given how much I had going on at that time — including my upcoming move back east to get married — I hoped I might be able to just monitor this for a few months to see if it went away.

Soon thereafter, I called Tomas, so we could brainstorm about what to do — he specializes in infectious diseases. He suspected I'd probably picked up something in India. He thought it was most likely not a cancer but what is called a "reactive node." He said he sees a lot of these in his practice. Plus, there was no history of cancer in my immediate family. I lived a healthy, balanced life. I'd been a vegetarian for more than 30 years. I exercised regularly. I didn't smoke, and probably drank two or three alcoholic beverages a year.

He did agree that lymphoma was a possibility, even though he thought it was less likely than our theory that the swollen nodes were due to an infection. Lymphoma comes in two main varieties: aggressive and indolent. With the more slowly growing ones, Tomas said, doctors sometimes decide, as is common in prostate cancer, to "watch and wait" before doing anything.

Tomas thought my plan to monitor the node was reasonable. If it grew, I'd need to act. Instead, over the ensuing months, the node shrank. A year later, it felt about half its original size. I'd never seen a cancer do that without treatment. I pretty much forgot about it.

When I first met Dr. Morrison, the ENT surgeon, I told him about the enlarged lymph node from two-and-a-half years earlier. He believed that it could not possibly be related to my tonsil cancer, since the node had shrunk. That's also what made me think that the node wasn't cancer. But that node's location on the right side, just beneath the angle of my jaw, is precisely where one of three nodes lit up on my PET scan.

My theory is that the lymph node my fiancée discovered that day in bed had already been invaded by cancer that had metastasized from my tonsil — and that it shrank because I was living such a healthy lifestyle. That idea seemed preposterous to Dr. Morrison. And when I told him at that same visit that my nodes and tonsil had shrunk while I was in India, he didn't buy that either.

As it would turn out, swollen lymph nodes were going to make another appearance in my life before my cancer would be diagnosed.

In the spring of 2016, I had just settled into a beautiful house in the Hudson River Valley, near Rhinebeck. The house was surrounded by woods, and out back was a pond graced by herons and a one regal swan. This retreat into nature felt like a balm to my wounded heart. My wife and I had split up three months before.

On my daily hikes I saw beaver, deer, fox, and even a toddler-sized bear cub one day. Upon spotting me, it ran straight up the side of a tree faster than I would have believed possible. After a split second I realized what I was looking at and, fortunately unmolested by the mother bear, I made a beeline the few hundred yards to my back door. After that, I started carrying a canister of bear-repelling pepper spray on my hikes.

But smaller creatures proved to be the bigger threat. In June, I developed the first of what would be three episodes of Lyme disease that summer. In each case, it started with a small, itchy, raised area on my skin that I thought might be a mosquito bite. But I knew I was in an area that was overrun with Lyme ticks. I had found both deer ticks, which carry Lyme, as well dog ticks, which don't, on my pant legs after hikes. One time I caught a deer tick climbing up the skin of my thigh.

In each instance of Lyme, the spot doubled in size by the next day and started to show a reddish border with a lighter color more centrally — a highly suggestive sign, though it hadn't yet progressed to the classic bull's-eye rash. By then, the rashes also hurt when I scratched them, as if the underlying tissue had been damaged. I got on the antibiotic doxycycline by the third day each time and quickly improved. The long-term and potentially devastating complications of Lyme almost always happen to people who don't get treatment early.

In July, on the second day of my second episode, I noticed lymph nodes on the right side of my neck had become enlarged and tender. Since this happened during an acute infection with Lyme disease, I assumed that was the cause. When I consulted with Tomas, he thought the nodes might have reacted because the Borrelia burgdorferi spirochete, a corkscrew-shaped bacteria-like organism that causes Lyme, spreads throughout the entire bloodstream soon after the infection begins.

After my second bout of Lyme, I continued to feel

well, but I noticed something unusual. For about a month straight, my tongue had been coated with a beige-colored film. I had spotted the coating because I follow the Ayurvedic hygiene recommendation of scraping my tongue every morning with a small hand-held implement designed for this purpose. I'd seen a coating like this for a day or two now and then in the past, but never so persistently.

Standing at the bathroom mirror in early August, I pointed a flashlight toward my mouth and investigated my tongue. What stood out, though, was my left tonsil. It was enlarged, from what I could see, to maybe half an inch, and was tinged grey. The right one looked normal. I didn't know what the cause was, but I was concerned. I'd seen thousands of enlarged tonsils in my years of practicing medicine, but never only on one side. I texted Tomas a photo. He didn't think much of it.

I knew that lymphomas could cause enlarged lymph nodes and swelling of lymphoid tissue like the tonsils. Online, I learned of another possibility — a primary cancer of the tonsil with metastases to the neck — a diagnosis I'd never seen when I was practicing medicine. But one aspect of my case spoke against tonsil cancer: my nodes were on the opposite side of the neck from the enlarged tonsil. Usually, when a tonsil cancer spreads, it goes to the nodes on the same side.

Tomas's and my ignorance about tonsillar cancer put us in good company. It appears that most physicians at the time of my diagnosis were unaware of the disease. The two primary doctors I consulted, both good clinicians, had been clueless, though one had been concerned about the nodes and lobbied me to have them biopsied. A dentist I spoke with, who prides himself on his careful oral exams to screen for cancerous and precancerous changes, hadn't heard of tonsillar cancer. A few years earlier, I'd read about the case of the actor Michael Douglas who had been diagnosed with HPV-related "throat cancer," but I hadn't remembered the details.

––––––––––––

In early November, when my lymph nodes were still enlarged two months after my third bout of Lyme disease, I decided to go in for tests. On an ultrasound and a later MRI — two non-invasive tests I'd insisted on starting with — the nodes looked abnormal, and possibly cancerous. The next step was a fine needle biopsy.

A physician's assistant (PA) at a local hospital in the Hudson River Valley did the procedure. I watched the image on an ultrasound monitor as the needle slid in and out. The PA maneuvered, trying to coax samples of two of the nodes into a small plastic syringe. None of this was painful other than the sting from the local anesthetic. The nurse kept a gloved hand on my shoulder the whole time and I was surprised how soothing that felt.

The PA filled one syringe after another with thick yellowish material that resembled a processed cheese product. Sitting in the corner of the room with a microscope, a pathologist checked the samples. Surprisingly, she found no cancer cells, and in fact, no cells at all, just dead tissue. I wasn't sure what to make of this result. The remnants of destroyed cells were a sign that a battle had been fought, but no enemy was found. Maybe it wasn't cancer.

After we were finished, the PA suggested that this could be good news: it could be a sign that my immune system was fighting whatever it was I had. That made sense to me. I learned a few weeks later that those nodes were indeed cancer. The biopsy hadn't been able to prove that, probably because there was a lot more dead stuff in the nodes than viable cancer cells. Months later, I went back over the events in my mind and saw a logic that had eluded me. I remembered something I'd read.

Back in the late 1800s, a physician at New York Hospital named William Coley was intrigued by reports of cancers that went into remission after the patients had recovered from serious infections. He wondered whether the invading bacteria had stimulated their immune systems, which then attacked the tumors. When he researched the question, he found over 45 cases in which tumor regressions were linked to infections.

He began experimenting on an Italian immigrant named Zola. Mr. Zola was a drug addict, near death, with an egg-sized malignancy on his right tonsil that was considered incurable. With his permission, Coley injected the streptococcus bacteria — linked to the potentially life-threatening skin infection erysipelas — directly into the tumor. After several attempts, Zola became infected. Immediately afterwards the mass started to shrink. Within two weeks it had disappeared.

Could something like what happened to Zola have happened to me, too? The antibodies my body made in response to my first infection with the Lyme bacteria would have been mobilized even more strongly one month later, when the bug was detected again. That's when my nodes got hot and tender. Because my immune system was so revved up by the Lyme, I figure it pounced on the cancer as well. It probably did so again when I got the third bout of Lyme. That's why the biopsy two months later found only dead cells.

The streptococcus toxin that Coley used was later modified to make it less dangerous, and it became "Coley's Toxin," which was used in cancer care for decades thereafter. Coley's Toxin met with with some success,

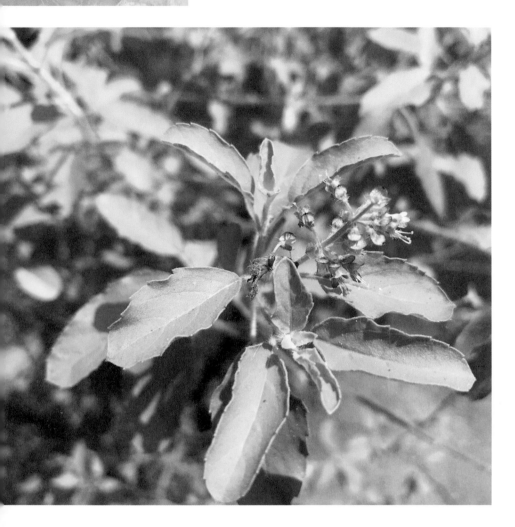

though it was never fully embraced by the medical establishment. Recent years have seen the rise of a new class of cancer drugs, which like Coley's Toxin stimulate the body to fight cancer, rather than attacking the cancer directly.

It was just such a drug that cured Jimmy Carter's cancer. The former president faced what seemed like terminal diagnosis: the deadly skin cancer malignant melanoma had spread to his liver and brain. Standard treatments available at that time almost always failed. But he lucked out — an experimental drug, Keytruda (pembroli-zumab) became available right when he needed it. After four months on the drug, Carter announced to the world that he was cancer-free.

Cancer cells have evolved strategies to evade immune detection and attack, so they can grow unchecked. You might say that drugs like the one Carter received turn off cancer's "invisibility cloak." Once his immune system was activated in this way, his cancer didn't stand a chance. Many believe that these new immunotherapy drugs are the biggest cancer-care advance in a generation. So far, only a few such drugs have been released but many more are, as they say, "in the pipeline." These drugs are tri-umphs of reductionist science, even though they don't always work and their sky-high prices and troublesome side effects are problematic. Their discoverer, James P. Allison, PhD, of the MD Anderson Cancer Center, was awarded the 2018 Nobel Prize.

None of my doctors recommended immunotherapy drugs, but they can't be faulted for that. Those that were available at the time were less effective than the chemo-radiation I ended up choosing. Interestingly, the repeated Lyme infections I suffered may have had the same kind of stimulating effect on the immune system. If I do end up cured, these infections may deserve some of the credit. Even if that's not so, the swollen nodes meant the cancer was diagnosed earlier than it might otherwise have been.

All I knew after the biopsy was that something was wrong, and that it might be cancer. I needed to know for sure. My ENT doctor at the time recommended we biopsy the tonsil, and since I agreed with him that metastatic tonsil cancer was the most likely explanation, we sched-uled it. I had hoped this procedure could be done in his office, but because of the risk of bleeding, he insisted on general anesthesia. This time, the test gave a definitive result: moderately differentiated squamous cell carcinoma caused by HPV.

Did stress cause my cancer? This turns out to be controversial — and demonstrates a major divide between doctors and patients. Most doctors are skeptical of a stress-cancer link; the scientific support for the notion is considered weak. But if you ask many cancer patients why they got the disease, stress is often the first thing they'll name.

The possible connection comes to mind when I think of my mother's sister, Helen. I actually had two Aunt Helens, both nuns. Back then, it was expected that devout Catholic families would send at least one child into either the convent or priesthood. Sister Helen Dolores, the baby of Mom's siblings, was on the brink of taking her final vows when she had a breakdown. She went bawling to the Mother Superior to tell her she couldn't go through with her vows, but according to Mom, Helen wasn't permitted to back out. She'd been miserable in the convent — a PhD in history scrubbing the rectory floors — and finally left toward the end of her life. While the stress-cancer connection is unproven, it's noteworthy that she developed five different primary malignancies in adulthood, including a rare blood cancer.

Of course, seen holistically, everything is multifactorial. Even though HPV is listed as the official "cause" of my cancer, why did I not clear the infection as most other people do? Why did the cancer manifest at the time it did, and not five years later or five years earlier? Why did my cancer seem to grow much more slowly than usual? Why did it, on more than one occasion get smaller without any medical treatment? That's wasn't normal for any cancer I'd ever seen.

There is an increasing recognition that stress can lead to inflammation — and inflammation has been linked to a growing number of cancers, including those caused by HPV. Perhaps even more importantly, being stressed leads many people to abandon good habits like going to the gym or taking a walk in nature in favor of scarfing junk food, binge-watching TV, smoking cigarettes, and drinking more alcohol than they should. The net effect is almost certainly an increase in any number of cancers.

I suspect the difficulty medical science has in making the link to cancer is that stress is hard to measure. Despite efforts to quantify it, the most accurate way to measure someone's stress levels is to simply ask them. But doctors are scientists. They want hard numbers, not subjective feelings. A bigger issue is that by the time a cancer has been diagnosed, it's often been slowly growing for years, if not decades. At what time should scientists measure stress levels to make the link? Nobody knows.

In my case, the critical time might have come 30 years ago. For the three years I was a medical resident I had enormous job stress, often working more than 100 hours per week and every third or fourth day on all-night-call in the hospital as part of a 36-hour shift. I was chronically deprived of sleep.

This could have been significant as this is around the time that Dr. Clark speculated that I may have been infected with HPV. Since that time, studies have linked sleep deprivation and overnight shift work to higher rates of developing cancer. I wonder whether the effects on my immune system from years of inadequate sleep might be the reason why a viral infection that most people clear spontaneously resulted, in my case, with viral genes infiltrating the DNA in my tonsil and later causing cancer.

At the end of my three years of post-graduate medical education, I had big black half-moons under my eyes. I assumed that was just what I looked like — until, three months later, as I rested and studied for my board exam, the black crescents disappeared. During residency, I'd been on nasal sprays and antihistamines for allergies so bad that I would sometimes sneeze 30 times in a row. That may sound funny, but it's painful. Once I finished my training, I never needed those medicines again. I also stopped the antacids I took for reflux, and the sleeping pills.

During the months before I was diagnosed with cancer, my stress levels had to have been high, despite my yogic lifestyle. If you look at those charts that assign points to stressful life events, I chalked up a bonanza in short order. I lost my marriage, to the person I thought was my best friend. Lost the dog I fed and walked in the woods every day. Lost the yoga studio where I had taught workshops and classes, which my ex decided to close while I was in India trying to figure my life out.

I also lost my financial stability when my wife closed the yoga studio. The workshops I planned to teach there were supposed to be my major source of income for the coming year — and one I couldn't quickly replace. That loss only added to the financial difficulties the marriage had brought. Moreover, because I hadn't seen the split coming, it took me a while to figure out where I would live, so I effectively became homeless. Before I left for India, all my possessions went into storage for the first time in my life. The house I moved into in the Hudson River Valley was furnished, so I only moved in a few things in with me. It felt to me as if I'd spent the entire year before my diagnosis living out of a suitcase.

I'll never know for sure what role stress played in

causing my cancer. But is it just a coincidence that my diagnosis came the year after my marriage unexpectedly fell apart?

———————

Yoga teaches that events we consider unfortunate, and react to negatively, may turn out to have an unexpected silver lining. I thought getting Lyme disease three times in one summer was an unalloyed negative, but actually, it may have saved my life.

The *Bhagavad Gita*, the most beloved of all Indian spiritual texts, teaches that each of us should align our efforts with some greater purpose — whatever we construe that to be. That's the key to finding fulfillment. Our attention should be on following our path with integrity and dedication — and not on what happens as a result. If your level of contentment rockets up and down in response to how you perceive events, or how others react to you, you are guaranteed a life with much suffering. That's because the universe and other people have a nasty habit of failing to comply with our wishes. The yogi aims for the middle path, avoiding both the extremes of elation and dejection.

"Skill in action" is the *Gita*'s definition of yoga. It's yogic to use your life and struggles to learn and grow, turning seemingly bad events into something that serves you. Yoga teaches that it's possible through your actions to change some bad karma into good karma. Focus not on whether you like what is happening, yoga teaches, but on what you are going to do about it.

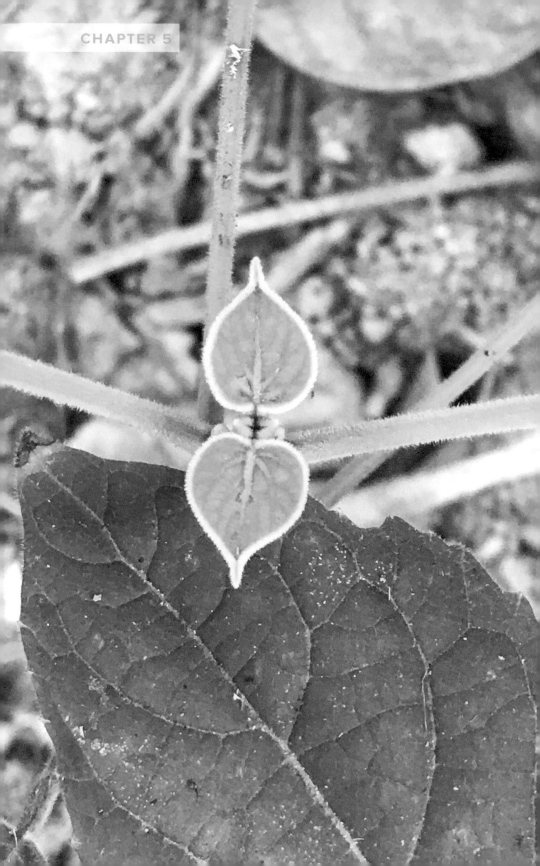

CHAPTER 5

"When the student is ready,
the teacher appears."

— Unknown

ZEN TENNIS

It was a blazing hot day the summer after my freshman year of college. I was playing tennis on the hard courts in Washington Park, in the finals of the Milwaukee County Parks 18-and-under tournament. A small crowd was watching, including a guy named John, who owned two tennis pro shops in town.

After I won, John approached me. "Would you be willing to feed me some balls so I can work on my shots in exchange for free lessons?"

This was an offer I could not refuse. I knew John from the pro shop. He had sold rackets to my father and me. At one time, he was the top-ranked tennis player in Wisconsin. He'd gotten good at tennis, partly because his parents' home was directly across the street from the Washington Park courts. That's why he was there the day of the finals.

"You're the only one of the guys in the tournament who uses his head on the court," John said. I'd been reading books on strategy and I guessed it was paying off. "I've seen your father play and thought he was an a**hole and always assumed you were, too."

A week later, we met for my first tennis lesson in Milwaukee's Lake Park, near my house. Early on in that session, John asked me to stand in the doorway of the fence that surrounded the courts. He had me wait in what's known as "the ready position," knees bent, looking straight ahead, racket poised in front of me — preparing to turn in either direction for an oncoming ball. We had been working on volleys, that is, balls struck on the fly.

John had been telling me what I already knew: you are not supposed to take your racket back on a volley. Instead, the proper technique is to meet the ball out in front of your body and punch it — which it what I thought I was doing. He tossed a ball toward my forehand side. As I prepared to strike it, the head of my racket smacked into the cyclone fence to the side of the opened door. This was an exercise in increasing my awareness of what I was actually doing. I got it instantly.

John told me I should buy a book called *The Inner Game of Tennis* and start reading it before our next get-together. He gave me a total of six lessons over a couple of months, using the methods the book advocated. It revolutionized my game. He taught me topspin on both the forehand and backhand, which I picked up quickly. My two-handed backhand — which I had modeled on Tony's — went from a relative weakness to a reliable weapon. John was a master teacher. I'm sure by simply watching the tournament, he had figured out most of what he wanted to teach me — long before we ever stepped on the court together.

I found the techniques described in *The Inner Game of Tennis* to be valuable beyond the game. Any time I wanted to teach myself a new skill, I used the methods described by the author, Timothy Gallwey. That book didn't just transform my tennis game; it had a huge impact on my entire life.

A few years ago, I got curious about the book. I remembered how much it had influenced me as an 18-year-old, but I couldn't remember the book itself, so I picked up a copy. The book differentiated the ego and the embodied mind, and described what Gallwey called "felt sense," a kind of inner awareness. The ego, he asserted, tries to control the show and often gets in the way of accomplishing what you hope for.

Gallwey talked about cultivating non-judgmental awareness and observing your habit patterns of body and mind. He taught methods of modeling the new habit patterns that you were attempting to develop. He also emphasized the importance of regulating the breath as you practiced and played the game.

As I re-read it, I found myself thinking, *Holy sh*t! It's a yoga book!* Even though Gallwey never used the word yoga once, the principles he espoused were all now familiar to me. And as I rediscovered, the book is dedicated to Guru Maharaj Ji, who was a teenage "born yoga master" at the time the book was published. This cherubic boy — who toured the West against his widowed mother's wishes — was ridiculed in the press for his fondness of ice cream and squirt guns, but he had thousands of devoted followers, including Gallwey, who considered his spiritual teachings to be transformational.

The methodology *The Inner Game of Tennis* described for changing the mind and body is almost identical to what I teach in my yoga therapy workshops to this day. Re-reading the book, I came to understand that I had not started practicing yoga at the age of 38, as I had assumed, but 20 years earlier. For the first 20 years, tennis strokes were my yoga poses.

Inner tennis was the doorway to understanding my body and mind in a way I never had before. As much as his approach improved my tennis game, it was this self-study — a cornerstone of the practice of yoga — that was truly revolutionary for me. I learned about myself on and off the court, especially my "shadow" side, which lay beneath my everyday awareness. This shadow was my desire to control what happened. To look good in other's eyes. I saw my subterranean insecurities. My deep-seated fear of failure. How wanting something badly can get in the way of achieving it. The latter lesson, I would need to keep relearning again and again.

I made one huge mistake at the time, though. I decided I could ignore all of Gallwey's suggestions about using the breath to further the process of the inner game. It didn't sound important to me, but I now see it as the crucial ingredient in yoga. I'm still trying to catch up with what I missed.

There is a common saying in the yoga world: When the student is ready, the teacher appears. It's been attributed to everyone from the Buddha to Lao Tzu, the author of the *Tao Te Ching*, but its actual origin is obscure. The teacher who appeared in my life was John, who mentored me in tennis. My guess is he didn't have any idea either that what he was transmitting was yoga. Gallwey must have known, though I'm not sure if he has ever acknowledged it publicly, other than indirectly by dedicating the book to Maharaji.

My next teacher, Patricia Walden — this time someone who was an actual yoga teacher — came into my life in 1995, when I started taking classes with her in Cambridge, Massachusetts. I had no idea that a chance encounter with a woman at a party who recommended Patricia's studio to me would change the course of my life. I was also unaware that Patricia was one of the most famous and most respected yoga teachers in the country.

I remember an evening in January 1997. I'd just come home from the urgent care center where I worked, and was sitting at the kitchen table. I was exhausted physically and emotionally. For months, I had been noticing that the tie I wore to work was feeling tighter around my neck. Not that this had anything to do with my cancer — I think it was just the way my inner self was trying to get my attention.

Corporations were taking over health care in Massachusetts, and in that environment, even the non-profits were putting money first. There was mounting pressure

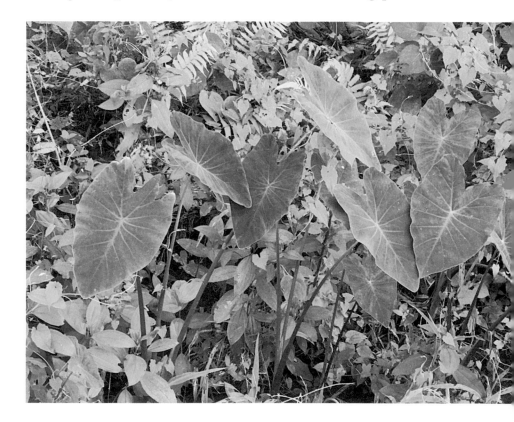

from higher ups to spend less time with each patient. In the clinic, I felt as if I was in that episode of *I Love Lucy* in which Lucille Ball frantically tries to wrap pieces of candy into individual wrappers as the conveyor belt moves faster and faster.

I had set high standards for the practice of medicine in a book I had published in 1995, *Examining Your Doctor*, but with less time to devote to each patient, I felt I couldn't live up to those standards. Getting to know patients, educating them about their health conditions, doing a thorough physical exam — all the parts of medical practice I found most rewarding — weren't viewed as important by the bean counters. What the HMOs saw as inefficiency, I saw as essential.

As I began to unwind that night in Cambridge, a thought bubbled up: *You don't have to do this anymore. What if you just write?* My writing career had been going well and I figured I could stop practicing medicine and I'd be okay.

As big a step as it would be, within 10 minutes I knew it was right. I called my mother to tell her what I'd decided. She laughed. A contrarian herself, she liked it when people bucked the system. It took me another six months to extract myself from my practice, but it was one of the best decisions I've ever made. I'll never know whether this epiphany was related to my growing inner awareness, but it came almost exactly two years after I started studying yoga with Patricia.

Practicing yoga built my capacity for both inner and outer awareness. As I continued to work with Patricia, I developed the ability to feel what was happening in my body with greater sensitivity. Knowing where a body part — say, the left index finger — is in space even without looking is the "felt sense" that Gallwey wrote about, something known as proprioception. Identifying subtle sensations inside the body, like feeling the heart beating, is the other part of "felt sense" — interoception. Yoga improves both.

With continued practice, my felt sense became progressively sharper. Masters develop heightened perceptive abilities, and this includes being able to "read" the state of the autonomic nervous system (ANS). For example, a yogi might detect subtle stress, mediated by the sympathetic nervous system, which would escape most people's awareness. Yogis can also calm the ANS, far more deeply than most people do when they relax.

In the year 2000, about five years into my explorations of hatha yoga and holistic healing, I began to see a traditional Japanese medical practitioner. I met the man I'll call Hiroyuki through friends. He'd moved to the Boston area to study public health. He was, as I recall, a 15th generation healer, who had learned from his mother and father at their clinic in Japan.

In our work together, Hiroyuki began the sessions, as is traditional among Japanese healers, by palpating my abdomen. He was feeling for abnormalities in the flow of chi. Chi (also written as qi and ki) means "life force energy," and is analogous to prana. Without my telling him anything, he would push one place and say, "This hurts, right?" and he was always correct. Other times, he might ask whether I had a mild ache with pressure, and again he'd be accurate.

Then he'd begin his work, using shiatsu, an acupressure massage, on my back; and moxibustion, the burning of medicinal herbs over acupuncture points on my arms, legs, and torso. Afterwards he'd retest the same spots in the abdomen and all the tenderness would be gone.

Around that time, I'd begun a two-year teacher training program in Iyengar yoga led by Patricia, who by then had been my teacher for five years. This was when I made a full-time leap into yoga. I was no longer seeing patients, though I kept my medical license. Instead, I began practicing yoga three or four hours per day. I read books on yoga, books on alternative medicine, and did research by investigating traditional holistic healers like Hiroyuki. I began to see him weekly.

One afternoon, during my home yoga practice, I made a breakthrough. Patricia had repeatedly suggested in class that I try to open the area of my lower abdomen as I practiced simple backbends. Despite my efforts — and my pattern was always to push too hard — I could never get that area to budge.

But this day, the recalcitrant area released its grip, and the tissues connecting my pubic bone to the navel region became more spacious. There was a feeling of warmth in my lower belly, even a slight burning sensation when I arched my spine backward. Given how limited my spinal movements were at that time, I should say as I moved *in the direction* of arching backward. My task then was not to bend backward per se, but to bring my chronically slouching posture in the direction of being upright by any amount.

Early the following afternoon, in my weekly appointment with Hiroyuki, I didn't initially mention this breakthrough. He took my pulse, using the technique that had been handed down to him, which was different from the one I'd learned in medical school, and different from what I would learn years later in Ayurveda. For the last year, he said, the region of the pulse that corresponded to the area between the pubic bones and the navel had been consistently imbalanced. Today it was good. He did mention that the area corresponding to my right upper back was still abnormal.

A few hours later, I was in a church basement in Cambridge for Patricia's dinner-time class. Early on, Patricia stood in her spot in the front of the room as the students assumed Triangle pose. "Timothy, look at you!" she said, motioning toward my abdomen. Then the stern taskmaster returned, "Now move your right scapula into your rib cage."

This was a moment of epiphany. Yoga, with its prana and chakras, was describing the same reality as Asian medicine with its meridians and chi. And in this case, there was clearly an anatomical correlate. By stretching the muscles and the connective tissue of the lower abdomen in a new way during my yoga practice, I had freed the "energetic blockage" that Hiroyuki had earlier diagnosed on pulse examination. And both systems detected an abnormality in my right upper chest — though it would take me another two years to figure out that that was related to the fall out of a window I'd suffered as a kid.

During my first trip to India, in 2002, I stood in the lobby of Kabir Baug, a yoga therapy center in Pune. The director, Dr. SV Karandikar, was a family physician turned yoga therapist. He asked me to come into a forward bending pose. I was not expecting this. I was there to observe the work he and his teachers did on several inpatients and hundreds of outpatients each week, not to be treated myself.

With my legs straight, I bent forward but as usual didn't get too far. My fingertips hovered several inches off the ground. When Dr. Karandikar saw the results, he said he wanted to get an X-ray of my spine.

"Why do you want to do that?" I asked.

"Because for someone who's been doing yoga as long as you have, that's not normal."

I was 45 years old and had no idea there was anything wrong with my spine. I knew that I was what I jokingly referred to a "remedial yoga student," because my body was so stiff. I figured that was from years of playing tennis, riding a bicycle, and never stretching. When I played sports, I had two speeds: on and off.

To get the X-ray of my spine, I made my way a few blocks over to a storefront clinic on Laxmi Road, a bustling shopping district in Pune. Seeing the modest setup and the antiquated equipment, I worried that I might get an overdose of radiation — but when I saw the films, I felt reassured. They were what doctors call "under-penetrated," meaning less radiation than optimal. It turned out Dr. Karandikar had specified they be shot that way. It helped him read soft tissue details that physicians back home don't try to assess from plain X-rays.

The film showed crescent-shape calcifications linking several of my upper back vertebrae to each other. The X-ray taken from the front revealed what Indians call bamboo spine. Dr. Karandikar gave me my diagnosis in Western medical terms: ankylosing spondylitis (AS). That's an autoimmune condition that causes debilitating stiffness and pain as the spinal joints fuse.

Clearly something was going on, and his diagnosis would explain my limited spinal movements in every plane. I was a longtime yoga student who couldn't bend forward or backwards well, or go into deep twists. But I was not convinced Dr. Karandikar's diagnosis was correct. The X-ray sure looked like AS, but I didn't have any of the pain that typically accompanies the disease, and I was older than most people are when diagnosed. There's

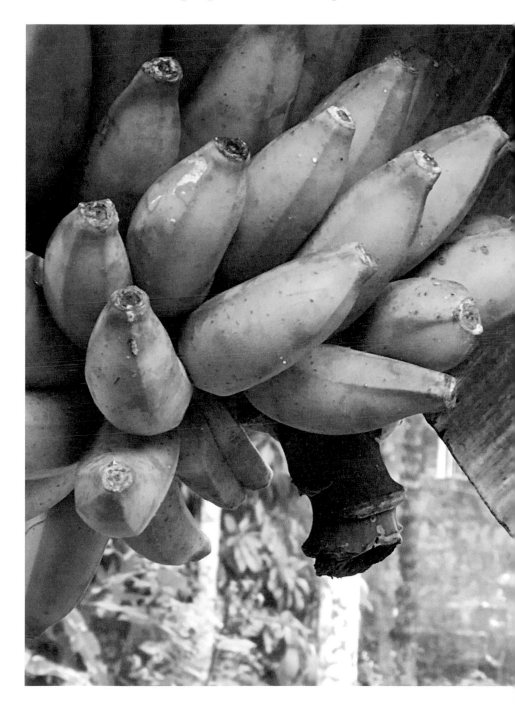

a genetic test for the disease, but when I returned to the States, I decided not to have it. I would leave as it an unanswered question.

Six months after Dr. Karandikar diagnosed this spinal condition, I was teaching alongside Patricia at a yoga conference in Colorado. Between our sessions, I was attending as many classes as I could fit in. I hadn't been sleeping well due to the altitude and was drained from all the strong yoga practices the teachers were leading.

The last day, I was about to begin a workshop on "Yoga for Injuries" with a teacher named Ana Forrest. All week in the cafeteria, I'd been hearing stories about how grueling her classes were. As I sat exhausted on my mat minutes before we started, it hit me that I might be making a big mistake.

Ana, a muscular woman with penetrating eyes, asked what injuries people had. "Knees?" Several arms went up. "Hips?" I raised my hand when she got to "upper back."

Ana didn't use a lot of props. She had us begin sitting cross-legged, without anything under the hips. There was no way I could sit in that position without rounding my back and collapsing my chest. She walked past my mat and spied my condition. She asked me to engage my lower abdominal muscles and relax my shoulders. I whispered to her that I had ankylosing of the thoracic spine. "It's like one functional unit," I said. "It doesn't really move."

She looked me straight in the eyes. "Well, it might move today."

"Actually," I told her, "it already has moved. When I started yoga, I was like this," I said, crooking my finger into an imitation of my pre-yoga posture, "and now I'm like this," I said, straightening my finger most of the way.

Her eyes twinkled.

Ana asked us to try to direct the breath to the area of our injuries. On perhaps twenty separate occasions over the course of the next two hours, she spent one to two minutes with me. She put her hands on my lower rib cage as I did Cobra pose, a gentle prone back arch. She coaxed me to change the way I was trying to open my chest. She encouraged me to not exert so much effort, and to move my spine at a slightly different angle than I'd been attempting. With her encouragement and hands-on guidance came new opening.

Afterward, as I walked out into bright sky against the backdrop of the Rocky Mountains, a warm afternoon breeze cooled the tears that streamed down my face. I didn't feel sad. I had a sense of release, a feeling that something had changed. I'd been doing yoga for years and seen many students cry in class, but nothing like it had ever happened to me.

———————

My first day back home after returning from the yoga conference, I was deep into a longer-than-usual yoga practice when it hit me. *I don't have ankylosing spondylitis. I know why my spine's the way it is. It's from the fall out the window!* The fall in question had occurred in the summer after fifth grade.

Immediately, I was certain this was correct. The doctor had cast my left wrist, fractured in six places, but I figured that I must have broken my spine, too. He must have missed those fractures. At some point down the road, my body must have fused all those joints together to protect me from damaging my spinal cord. That's what caused the bony bridges linking adjacent vertebrae visible on the Pune X-ray. It's not as if I'd suppressed the memory of the injury — I'd just never made the connection to my spine before.

So, this was the sequence: physical opening while practicing yoga, an emotional release, new understanding. To say this is something that wasn't covered in my medical school curriculum would be an understatement.

"The issues are in the tissues," yogis like to say.

The next day, I went online to try to learn more about Ana. I found an interview published in a yoga magazine. In it, she said, "I look at my students, and I can see where energy is blocked." Turning to her interviewer, Ana said, "For example, for you, one of the places your energy gets bogged down is around the throat, C6, T1. If I were to work with you, I'd go after that in poses, maybe unleashing a memory of falling out of a tree or somehow injuring yourself."

"I had a neck injury in 1992," the writer admitted.

I felt that what Ana was describing — seeing an energetic blockage, creating physical opening in the area, followed by understanding something that you hadn't before — was exactly what had just happened to me. I was glad I hadn't seen the article before I met her, or I might have worried that my expectations had influenced the outcome.

When I began yoga, I was not what yogis, dancers, and body workers would call "embodied." Despite my years of tennis, I didn't have a lot of bodily awareness. My posture was lousy, and I had no idea what good posture even was. Posture was never so much as mentioned in my medical education. If you want to see atrocious posture, head over to a hospital cafeteria and check out the shapes in the long white coats. Unbeknownst to me, I had become a member of a large and influential group of health care professionals that I call "Doctors without Bodies."

But after decades exploring yoga, bodywork, Ayurveda and other modalities, I have grown my bodily awareness to a high degree. As much as I respect the scientific method, I have come to believe that cultivated awareness is a valuable tool that can supplement — and sometimes if necessary, challenge — information that comes from studies. My increased ability to feel precisely what's happening in my body allows me to appreciate the effects of various treatments that I might have been oblivious to previously. It has guided me in every step of this cancer journey. It has also made a difference in how I dealt with the ruptured tendon in my quadriceps, which was the result of an accident I had shortly after my second case of Lyme.

That day, I was hiking the woods near a stunning Japanese garden. I slipped when I stepped onto a rock, still damp from morning rains. This was eight days before my divorce hearing and, as I would realize much later, it was the 10th anniversary of my mother's death. As I stepped, I watched my right boot slide back maybe an inch. I was able to right myself using the balancing skills that I'd gained by practicing yoga. I wasn't going to fall. But my back leg thought it would protect me by reflexively contracting as hard as it could. I felt a sharp pain just above my left knee, and then I fell over.

I'd torn the tendon of the body's biggest muscle, the quadriceps, right where it attaches to the kneecap. The operation to repair it would be the first surgery I'd ever had. On the advice of a friend from Rhinebeck, I'd chosen an orthopedic group in Albany, more than an hour north. My surgeon specialized in sports medicine, worked with local college teams, and did lots of knee operations.

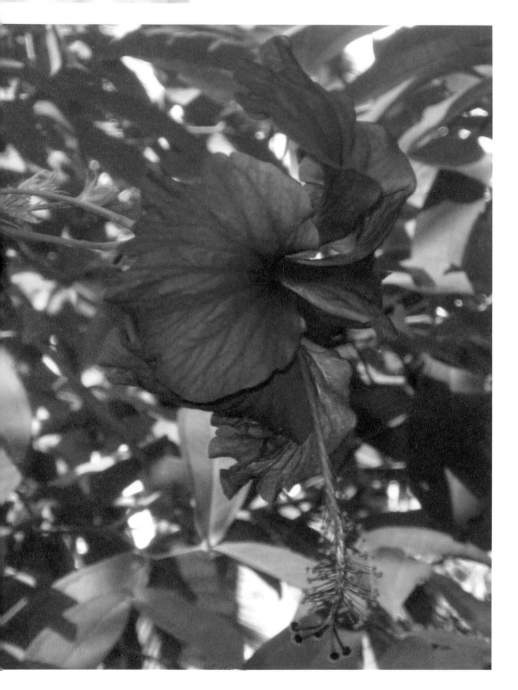

I chose to have a spinal block, because it's less risky than general anesthesia. Although the anesthesiologist suggested a drug to sedate me during the procedure, I asked to not be given it. I figured I'd rather be clear-headed throughout. I was able to speak with the surgeon a few times while he operated. He even pulled back the drape so I could see the torn tendon after he first opened the leg up. He did it again after he'd stitched the two ends of the tendon together. Seeing my before- and after-knee was surreal since I couldn't feel anything below the waist.

The lack of sedation meant that my post-anesthesia recovery was quick. Less than an hour after he closed the wound, I was discharged from the surgical facility. My friends Andy and Vicki had driven down from southern Vermont to take me to their place, which was where we'd decided was best for my recuperation. They lived in an old farmhouse and had set up an inflatable bed in the middle of the living room.

Right after the operation, the orthopedist placed a brace on my leg, mid-calf to mid thigh, with steel rods along the sides and Velcro straps securing it. It had a dial with which the doctors could precisely adjust the degree of flexion and extension of the knee joint. For the first six weeks after the operation, it was to be set at zero degrees. My leg would be straight all day and all night. When I heard this, I envisioned walking around like Frankenstein's monster.

But even before I left the surgery center, I noticed that with the dial set at zero, I could bend the knee 10–15 degrees. Thinking this couldn't be correct, I showed it to the surgeon. He assured me this was normal. I thought, wow, what the orthopedist calls zero degrees was to the yogi a whole lot more. And that extra mobility proved to be crucial.

For the first few weeks after the operation, the only rehabilitation exercise the surgeon had assigned was "quadriceps setting." I was supposed to contract my front thigh muscle isometrically, hold it for a few seconds, and then repeat it for a total of ten times. Three sets, two or three times per day. I thought, *That's it?*

I had already lost a lot of muscle. It's said that if the quadriceps muscles aren't exercised, they lose three percent of their mass every day. In the three weeks between the injury and the operation, mine would have shrunk more than 60 percent. I knew it would take many months to build the muscle back up. If I couldn't exercise it more than what they'd prescribed, I was worried that my thigh might atrophy further.

After my first night at Andy and Vicki's, I got out of the inflatable bed, and, on a whim, I decided to try Triangle pose. I found a place in an adjacent reading room, where old nails weren't poking through the floor planks as they were in the living room. Standing between Andy's Hofner bass guitar and the overstuffed armchair Vicki calls Teddy, after the former president, I separated my legs and turned my right foot to the side. As I exhaled, I hinged at the hip joint and lowered the right side of my torso toward my right leg, while rotating my rib cage to the left. It felt amazing. I changed to the other side, this time with the left leg in front. That side worked, too!

Then I tried balancing in Half Moon pose — lifting the back leg off the ground from Triangle. I was amazed that I was able to do that, too, and on both sides. Every time I inhaled, I bent both knees the 10–15 degrees the brace allowed. Every time I exhaled, I straightened the knee, but I never locked it. I could feel this was exercising my injured leg much better than quadriceps setting.

I didn't have the benefit of a study that examined the best yoga poses for the post-surgical recovery of quadriceps tendon ruptures. Unfortunately, there aren't any of those. Nor was I aware of any recommendation that had been passed on from yoga masters. I simply tried a few poses and saw how my body reacted. My body told me what it liked and didn't like. It let me know what was too much. And its feedback indicated what was likely to help.

Using my cultivated awareness, I designed my own protocol on the spot. As my strength grew — and then slowly over the weeks as the orthopedist adjusted the dial, allowing a greater flexion at the knee — I modified the routine as my body and breath dictated. This method of clinical decision-making is verboten in modern medical practice. It's not considered evidence-based (EBMers have decided that the direct feedback from the body does not constitute evidence). It's seen as subjective. It's not measurable. It can't be verified.

I declined the surgeon's offer for physical therapy. I figured I could do better on my own with yoga. I showed him a few of the poses I'd been practicing at our first post operative visit, and he was amazed. He could tell I knew what I was doing, and that my routine was safe. And he couldn't help but notice how quickly I was regaining function. He'd given me crutches, but within days I had stopped using them.

———

I use a similar process when I practice yoga therapy. I observe the students doing the practices I suspect might be good for them. Based on what I see and what they report, I have a very good idea of what's likely to serve them — and what won't.

I came up with the acronym SNAPS for the system I use to assess clients and plan their therapeutic routines. SNAPS stands for Structure, Nervous System and Breath, Ayurveda, Psychology, and Spirituality — the five general categories by which I map the holistic terrain of mind, body, and spirit.

Thus, as I evaluate a student — say, a woman with low back pain — I observe her posture as she sits, stands, and walks. I have her do various yoga poses, assessing them for symmetry and anatomical alignment. I observe her balance of effort and relaxation as she practices. I watch her breathe, looking for where, how, and how smoothly her body moves as she inhales and exhales. I gauge the state of her autonomic nervous, seeing if it is tipped excessively toward either the sympathetic or the parasympathetic side. Using a variety of techniques, including pulse diagnosis, I assess her Ayurvedic constitution and her current state of balance. I ask about her thoughts and emotions, her level of stress. I inquire if she has a sense of meaning in her life, some connection to something bigger than herself.

I am looking for imbalances in any of the dozens of areas that constitute the five SNAPS categories. Based on what I find, I'll craft a practice designed to help move her in a variety of ways back towards balance. Although I hope to help her back pain, I know that the best way to do that will depend on the specifics of her situation. For some people, improving their posture or their muscle strength or their flexibility would be the best method. Others need relaxation. Some folks harbor resentments, even suppressed rage, that might need to be excavated to relieve their pain. Many people suffering from low back strain need some combination of all these things for optimal healing.

In the seven months I lived in the Hudson River Valley, even before I hurt my leg, my yoga practice had become softer. With fiery pitta as part of my nature, I had pushed myself too hard in asana, pronounced AHS-suh-nuh, the Sanskrit word for the poses. I had held postures for a minute or longer, continually working to come more deeply into each position.

This is what yogis call "playing the edge." You come as deeply as you can into a pose, and attempt to go deeper by dint of will. The theory goes, you tug, tug, tug, and slowly you stretch the stubborn muscles as if they were Turkish Taffy, one of my second-tier childhood candies.

But in the last few years I've stopped doing this. Instead I play the edge by coming toward my maximum, in the case of a twisting pose like Triangle, on the exhalation. Then I move slightly away from my maximum on the inhalation. The next time I exhale, I again move deeper into the twist. This back and forth continues over several breaths. I call this process "pendulation."

I have found pendulation to be better for my nervous system, which has been overly activated since I was a kid. To my surprise, I discovered that with the lower degree of effort needed to pendulate, I go much farther into the poses — without causing the niggling injuries that I'd experienced with continual stretching at the edge. That method works, too — I did it for years — but for me pendulating in and out has been a breakthrough. It has also revolutionized how I teach asana.

My approach to aerobic exercise has undergone a similar change. When I got to Burlington after finishing my cancer treatment, I bought myself an elliptical machine on Craigslist. With its smooth gliding motion of the legs and arms, it seemed like the perfect way to continue to rehabilitate my leg after the quadriceps tendon rupture and to build back my stamina. They say that the fatigue can last a year once you've finished chemoradiation.

Years ago, when I first discovered ellipticals, I used to go for 45 minutes, working out at a high intensity. My heart rate would climb to the mid-140s, at the high end of the recommended aerobic range for my age. By the end, sweat was running down my temples. My shirt was stuck to my chest and back.

But as I got more into Ayurveda, I was won over by the ancient field's notions about exercise. Rather than there being an optimal amount or style of exercise for everyone — as modern medicine sometimes suggests — Ayurveda personalizes the approach based on constitution, overall health, and other factors. As always in Ayurveda, the correct approach for any condition is: it depends.

Since I have a good deal of pitta, I liked to work out hard, but Ayurveda says that's not what's best for me. I need to counteract my tendency to overdo — and look for slower and more soothing forms of exercise. Pittas should exercise just to the point where the brow becomes moist. They should avoid exercising outdoors in the midday heat. Activities like swimming, early morning walks, or hiking in the woods may be best. They provide pittas a good, balancing workout, and are much less likely to result in overheating. I ended up dropping my Y membership and starting hiking and dancing more.

Two weeks into my move to Burlington, and two months after finishing cancer treatment, I decide to try the elliptical machine for the first time. After a single minute on a low setting, I'm panting. I know I've had enough. My heart rate topped 150. The recommended high end for aerobic exercise at my age is about 135.

I let the machine sit for a few weeks and just dance for 15 or 20 minutes a few times per week, as my energy allows. By four months after I finished cancer treatment, I am dancing more like 40 minutes at a time. But now I want to step it up. Tomas, my med school friend, is coming for a visit soon, and he plans to bring his bicycle in the back seat of his convertible. We plan to renew an old tradition for us, and tour my new home town by bike, and I want to start to get in shape for that.

I try a homemade version of interval training. I dance for maybe 10 minutes and then get on the elliptical machine for a few minutes, dance some more and try the machine again. But my energy is up and down. I exercise one day, then don't feel up to it the next day or two, so I just rest.

And then I put it together — I had been pushing myself to exercise at a certain level of intensity, and it was too much. I had been imposing an idea of how much I thought I should be exercising at this stage of my recovery, rather than asking my body its opinion. That was my pitta talking, not my higher wisdom.

I try a different tack. Next time I get on the elliptical machine, I close my eyes, paying no attention to the timer. Without the visual input, I simply tune into my bodily sensations and focus on taking slow, nasal breaths. When I feel like it, I switch from striding forwards to backwards, and backwards to forwards. If I feel fatigue or any strain or if the breath becomes labored, I get off the machine and resume dancing.

The first time I try this more embodied style of interval training, I last one minute and 40 seconds. I'd been doing more than twice that amount. I dance for a while then get back on the machine. This time I make it two minutes and 25 seconds. The next time, I feel comfortable for four minutes and 15 seconds. And then a funny thing happens. I don't feel wiped out the next day. After that, I was able to exercise every day again — all because I'd listened to what my body had been trying to tell me.

I often feel uncomfortable when I read a story of a "heroic cancer" patient who runs a marathon or climbs Mount Everest. While I'm sure such achievements bring psychological rewards, I worry they might come at a cost. Exercise carried to an extreme can suppress the immune system. The idea of doing something extraordinary to triumph over cancer is just that: an idea. It comes from the head, the intellect. Doing it may require listening to the mind's directive, and overruling the body's feedback — exactly the mistake I'd made with the interval training.

I would need to make that mistake one more time: the bike tour of Burlington proved to be just another idea. Tomas, riding out in front, set a slower-than-usual pace, and we started out on relatively flat land. Still, after a mile or so, I started to realize that even that was too much. After we climbed a simple hill, I was panting and my heart pounded in my chest. I needed to stop and rest, and then turn back toward home.

I had found a better way to exercise in my experiments on the elliptical machine, not by consulting my doctors about how much I should be doing at that stage of recovery. I didn't consult the scientific literature either. Instead, I simply got out of the way, tuned into my body and breath, and they provided the answer — just as they had with the yoga program I'd devised to rehab my leg after surgery.

———————

I sort through the mountain of possessions in the Vermont lake house. The modest summer home had been in my family since the early 1960s. The plywood A-frame, which my mother had built to her specifications for a few thousand dollars, gave a splendid view of the lake. It was located on an acre of land that Mom had bought for $1000, and which adjoined my grandfather's property.

Mom had figured out an ingenious way to wind a road down her father's land on the steep side of the valley, to access lakefront that had long been considered inaccessible. For many years, ours was the only house on that side of the lake. That stunning piece of land, right next to a brook with a small waterfall, was regarded as almost worthless before Mom cracked the puzzle. For the second time in my life, my mother had materialized a home that, theoretically, we should not have been able to afford.

I loved that place, nestled in the woods, but I rarely had a chance to use it. I'd been trying to sell it for years, but never received a single offer until the week after I finished chemoradiation. I accepted it immediately. Now I'm trying to rescue all the family photos and other memorabilia before the sale closes.

I uncarth a trophy with a golden tennis player perched on top of a marble pedestal — his knees bent, his back arched, up on his tiptoes, as he prepares to strike a serve. Both of his arms are raised. There's a ball poised on his left fingertips, but his right hand is empty, the golden racket long since gone.

I read the inscription. It's my prize for winning the Milwaukee County Parks tournament — the event that brought John and, as I would later discover, yoga into my life. Leaving the other trophies behind, I bring the memento to my new home in Burlington, and place it on top of the bookcase that holds blankets, bolsters, and blocks in my yoga practice space.

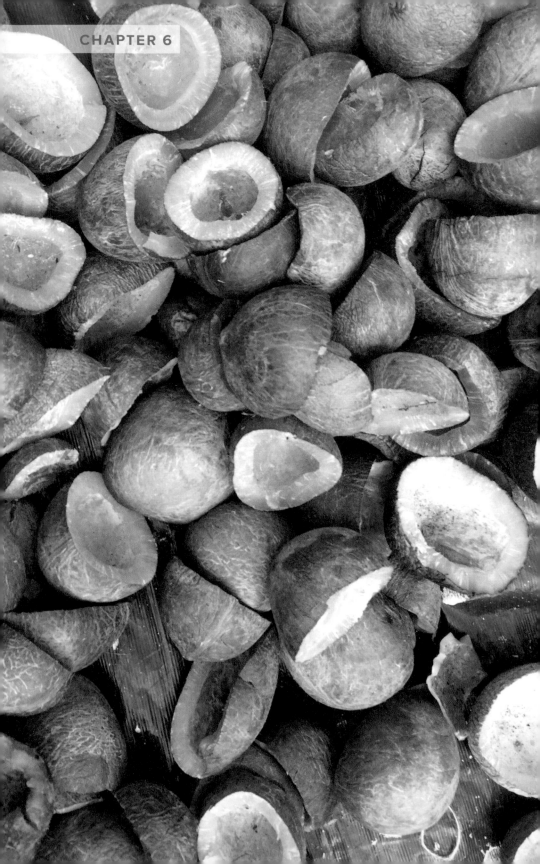

CHAPTER 6

"Foolish is the doctor who dismisses
the knowledge of the ancients."

— Hippocrates

SHAM ACUPUNCTURE?

In 1995, I began taking yoga classes with Patricia Walden
in Cambridge, Massachusetts. I had only the vaguest
idea of what I was getting myself into. I had some inkling
it might be good for my body and mind, but I was also
very much there for the spirituality. What I hadn't expected was that yoga would be so intellectually stimulating — and endlessly interesting to me. Yoga challenged
my mind at least as much as it challenged my body. And
it brought them together like never before.

About a year after I begun studying with Patricia, I
found that I had become fascinated with anatomical connections of the sort never taught in medical school. As
I did the poses, I started to notice a subtle chaining between parts of the body that I had never thought of as
having any interrelationship. Who knew that the little
toe is connected to the rib cage?

I wasn't calling it prana yet, but as I did asana, I was
able to follow the flow of energy between the bones and
the soft tissue. My awareness tunneled into my body. I
could sense the prana coursing through its tributaries,

penetrating its interwoven sheaves of muscle, bone, ligament and — the element that links them all, though I knew little about it at the time — the connective tissue, also called fascia.

This connective tissue is like the white parts of a grapefruit. Peel off the skin and the fruit is still round. Each section is surrounded by a thin membrane that holds its shape and separates it from its neighbors. If you break a section apart, you will see that each smaller piece is wrapped in yet another membrane. This is exactly what the fascia does in the body, enveloping the whole as well as the parts.

Five years into my love affair with yoga, I was hanging out with my brother Tony in his living room. I told him I'd discovered "that when I separate my fourth and fifth toes, I can bring more air into my lungs." It took me years of practice to get any opening between those toes, as if the muscles involved simply didn't work. Then one day, practicing at home in Boston, the little toe on the right foot woke up. From then on, I could separate it from its neighbor. The left little toe followed a few weeks later.

Tony looked at me, tipping his head to one side as his lips tightened, and said nothing. I took his expression to mean, *Whoa, time to get back to planet Earth*. And weird as this may sound to the uninitiated, I've talked to other yogis who've had exactly the same bodily experience. I suspect what's at work is the fascial web of connectivity between all the structures of the body.

Before yoga, I might not have known how to react to such claims as rib-toe connections any better than Tony. One of the things yoga has taught me is to suspend disbelief — or rather to put my trust in my own experience.

Undeterred by his skepticism, I offered to show Tony a yoga trick that might help with his chronically slumping posture. He agreed to try it. My brothers and I had the same slouching posture as our late father. My brother Ray calls it "chest on backwards."

When I started practicing asana, my head jutted a good six inches in front of my shoulders. I remember my sister Debbie's wedding reception at Milwaukee's lovely Estabrook Park, 20 years before this visit to Tony and Madelyn's house. My father and my two brothers sat at a picnic table, their spines tracing three question marks, the curves increasing in severity according to age. Looking at my father's spine, the worst of them all, I thought, *There's my future.* After years of yoga, my present has broken free of the future I once feared.

One of the most powerful techniques I used to change my spine came straight out of the Iyengar yoga toolbox. I decided to try it on Tony. I wrapped a yoga strap around his back, under his arms, and over the front of his shoulders, leaving the ends hanging down his back. Standing behind him, I crossed the straps and tugged the ends of the strap down, which pulled his shoulders blades back and down. His chest lifted, and he stood the straightest I've ever seen him.

Just then, Madelyn walked into the room, her thick auburn hair tied back. "Tony," she said, face brightening, "you look great!"

When I was back a year later, I spotted a blue yoga strap with a chrome buckle tightly coiled on Tony's desk. He never mentioned it and I never saw him use it — I don't even know if he bought it himself or if Madelyn got it for him — but I was impressed. Madelyn also mentioned that my nephew Jonathan, then 15, was using a neti pot to rinse his nasal passages, help for seasonal allergies. Yoga, it seemed, had found its way into their home — or at least had got its little toe in the door.

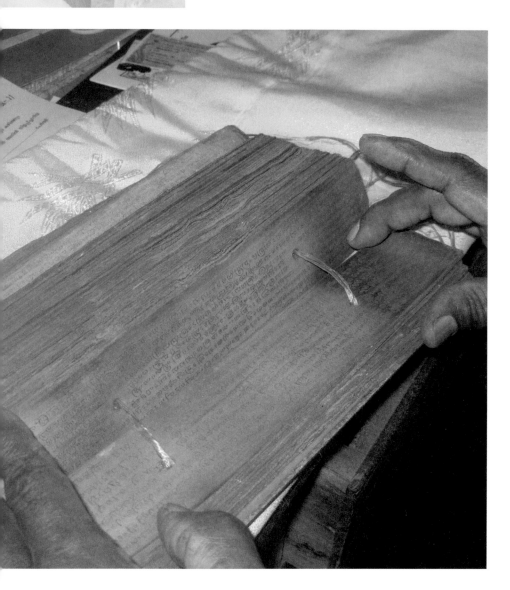

One hallmark of evidence-based medicine, as its name
suggests, is the value it places on empirical evidence: information acquired by direct observation via the senses or
by experimentation. Especially the latter. This is a value
it shares with Ayurveda and yoga. Ayurveda is an empirical science that has refined its theories and treatments

over the millennia — thousands of doctors over thousands of years meticulously observed the responses of millions of patients. Yogis spend years honing their powers of introspection. Indeed, the tradition teaches that no tool is more trusted than properly cultivated direct perception.

Over the course of their lives, masters of Ayurveda, like yoga masters, progressively refine their perceptive abilities. Their assessments can be both reliable and reproducible — qualities admired in science. But since their empirical evidence is not quantifiable, and has not been verified by the kind of rigid testing protocols that EBM insists on, much of it is summarily dismissed by physicians. This means that patients never even hear about potentially helpful treatments — like the turmeric-based skin cream I used to heal my radiation dermatitis.

Long before I went to medical school, I was skeptical of reflexology. That's the type of deep foot massage that proponents claim can both diagnose and treat a wide variety of illnesses. In college, I came across one of those laminated cards that show a diagram of the bottoms of the feet, with little cartoon renderings of the internal organs to which each spot on the sole supposedly corresponds. Press on the area at the ball of the foot, and you stimulate the stomach. A feeling of pain with pressure at that spot might indicate gastric trouble.

The notion that you could change the functioning of internal organs, or diagnose problems in those organs, by pushing on different areas of the foot sounded downright nutty to me. For comic relief, I'd pull that laminated card out of my wallet at parties. Mind you, I had never spent even one minute investigating reflexology. I'd just assumed, as most of my medical colleagues do to this day, that what sounded like baloney to me must be baloney and I didn't waste time checking it out. This was the same error *The Atlantic's* Dr. Hamblin made when analyzing alternate nostril breathing.

I hadn't thought about reflexology for a couple of decades when, during my first trip to India in 2002, I was offered a chance to learn about it. While I was studying yoga at BKS Iyengar's Institute in Pune, I got to know Allan, a Northern California yoga teacher and a long-time practitioner of reflexology. I was observing Allan and his wife, Jaki, who were assigned to guide a woman through a yoga therapy practice that Mr. Iyengar had developed for her.

One day, at lunch, Allan asked me how much I knew about reflexology. Not much, I told him. He said that if I were interested, he would be happy to give me a free session. By then I'd learned to take opportunities like this when they presented themselves. I didn't mention my former skepticism and decided to simply experience the session with an open mind. This is a yogic approach to the unknown: rather than simply asserting that something is true or not, a good teacher says, "Try this and see what you think." I was going to try a session of reflexology, and see what I thought.

Allan came to my tiny hotel room and we put the mattress directly on the floor — just enough room around it for him to work. He is not a big man, but his hands are vise-like. I soon realized that this was not going to be a soothing foot massage. It felt more like a trip to the dentist. Allan found spots on the soles of my feet that were remarkably tender, and pushed firmly.

I'd told him about my spinal condition, which I'd just learned about the week before. So when he pushed on the inside edge of each foot, and told me he could tell my spine was abnormal, I wasn't that impressed. Moving his focus over to the area that corresponds to the intestines, he asked if I'd been constipated lately.

Now that was interesting. Even though I almost never suffered from constipation back home, and tended more toward diarrhea when traveling in the developing world, I had indeed been constipated for the last few days. He told me that he sensed that I was dehydrated. I remembered that I'd been having trouble finding a refill for my water bottle, and had not been drinking as much as I should have been. But Allan didn't know about any of that.

He spent more than an hour on my feet. Even though the treatment was painful, when he finished my nervous system was deeply relaxed. Allan left and I spent the next fifteen minutes resting in Shavasana — the Corpse pose, in which you lie on your back, eyes closed, with your arms and legs splayed to the sides. I got up, took a few sips of water, walked to the bathroom, and had the most efficient, effortless, non-pathological, complete colonic evacuation of my life. More and more, intuition had been guiding my life, and now my gut was telling me that reflexology worked.

On a sunny morning during my second trip to India, I sat on the edge of a twin bed. 2005 had just turned to 2006, and I was at a small Ayurvedic center in rural Kerala. The place had been recommended to me by an Ayurvedic physician I'd recently met at another Ayurvedic institution — a famous hospital that had been disappointing to me. Dr. Swapna was on a rotation at that hospital as part of her postgraduate studies, but she was not affiliated with it. She told me that she came from an Ayurvedic family — they ran a center nearby. "We do things a little differently there," she said, and thought I might find it of interest. In particular, she raved about Jaypal, the center's massage therapist.

There was a knock on my open door. It was the center's managing director, a kind man named Balakrishnan, Dr. Swapna's uncle. He wore western slacks and a short-sleeve button-down shirt. With him at the door was a spry, elderly man with glistening eyes. He was dressed in a traditional dhoti, hanging down to his ankles, and a crisp, short-sleeve shirt. "This is Chandukutty Vaidyar. He's an Ayurvedic doctor, but he doesn't speak English. I've asked him to come see you."

This was the first I'd heard of this doctor, but I invited them in. Neither of them knew anything about my medical history, just that I was a physician from America interested in Ayurveda. Although Balakrishnan could have translated, Chandukutty had no questions. He pointed down at my feet and said, "Very healthy," in English. He had judged my overall state of health, just by looking at my feet.

Chandukutty walked over and sat on my right side. He lifted my wrist and placed the pads of his first three fingers on the pulse. Dr. Swapna had been teaching me pulse examination, and had stressed the importance of using the tips of your fingers, which have greater sensitivity than the pads. I had been spending five to 10 minutes just trying to get a basic pulse reading. Chandukutty left his fingers on my wrist for perhaps three seconds, and he was done. His eyes got big.

Next, he cradled my right arm in his and pushed on a spot near my elbow. I would later learn this was a marma point. It felt strange when he palpated it, like the vaguely electrical sensation you might get when an acupuncture needle is turned. Marma points, which are said to be energetic junctions, might be the historical precursors of acupuncture points — Ayurveda appears to be considerably older than TCM, and there was loads of contact between the ancient cultures.

Then he moved to the other arm. After Chandukutty pushed on the same marma point on my left elbow, the fire in his eyes again grew bright. He extended his arm around behind me, lifted my shirt, and placed his fingers directly on the area of my upper back damaged in my childhood injury. His physical exam lasted less than a minute, and yet he'd been able to pick up something that had eluded every conventional physician I'd ever seen.

"Stay for 30 days," Chandukutty Vaidyar said, "and we can cure your spine." I explained that I had a non-refundable plane ticket and couldn't stay that long. I had to fly in just over two weeks. My plan had been to use my remaining time to tour the backwaters of Kerala and visit the city of Mysore, a hotbed of yoga in the neighboring state of Karnataka.

"Fourteen days or we won't treat you."

"Okay," I said, "I'll stay for 14 days." I figured I could visit Mysore another time.

Jaypal massaged me every day with oils that Chandukutty had brought with him. After a few days, he began another treatment that Chandukutty had prescribed. This one, called Kati Basti, was aimed directly at my spine. As I lay on my stomach on the treatment table, Jaypal built a 6-inch ring of wet chickpea flour over my mid-to-upper back, which stuck up more than an inch from my skin. This treatment is typically prescribed for low back pain and applied to that area of the body, but my spinal fractures were in the middle of my back, so Chandukutty wanted it there.

Jaypal poured in warm oil into the central area, walled in by the wet flour like a moat. It felt delicious. Each time the oil began to cool, he spooned out some of it out and added oil he'd warmed. Each time the warm oil hit my skin, it felt so good, I couldn't wait till the next time he did it. Even the sound of the spoon as it scraped the steel bowl that held the warm oil became relaxing. This process continued for half an hour. Afterwards, he removed the dough, and I rested on the table.

Ayurveda believes that oils applied to the skin and allowed to soak in can penetrate deep into the body — even into the spinal bones — a claim unlikely to be taken seriously by western physicians. I couldn't help but notice, though, that the stubborn area of my upper spine gained more opening in 14 days with Chandukutty than in the 41 days I'd spent at the renowned Ayurvedic hospital. At that hospital, the care had seemed mass-produced, and of lower quality. It was as if they were trying to imitate allopathic medicine. The resulting hybrid, to my mind, wasn't nearly as good as the original.

I had been looking for an Ayurvedic doctor who practiced the art in a more traditional and authentic manner, and I was convinced that I'd found one in Chandukutty. My spine was bending backward further than it ever had. I still wasn't what anyone would call flexible, but the progress was encouraging. My last day, Chandukutty asked me if I would like to become his student. I felt honored. We decided I would return the following year to get treated, and then spend time shadowing him while he saw patients at his clinic.

While I was studying Sanskrit in Bangalore (now called Bengaluru) in preparation for returning to study with Chandukutty, I met a local Ayurvedic physician. He'd just opened a one-room storefront clinic. I walked in one afternoon when he wasn't busy, and introduced myself. I returned to visit a few more times.

We got talking one day and I asked about treating vata. I hadn't been sleeping that well in my room back at the Sanskrit academy. He suggested I rub sesame oil on my scalp, right where the skull bones come together above the forehead. This is the location of the anterior fontanelle, what's left of the soft spot that babies have, before the bones knit together.

There's a trick Krishna would later teach me to find this spot. You place the end of your thumb on the tip of your nose and reach up with the middle finger to the skull in the midline. There should be a slight depression there, but in my case there wasn't — the whole area felt rock-hard. In that case, the doctor said he wasn't sure the sesame oil would work, so I never tried it.

When I got to Kerala, I asked Chandukutty about my lack of a palpable fontanelle. I had read that in Ayurveda it's viewed is a portal through which excess pitta escapes the body. Its being blocked in my case might mean too much heat would be retained in my brain, which could lead to inflammation or other problems later on.

Chandukutty said he would bring medicine for that on his next visit. Soon, just before bed one evening, Jaypal arrived at my door cradling a steel bowl with a spoon handle protruding from it. Inside was a dark-chocolate-colored salve, tarry in consistency and with a strong organic smell, not unpleasant but weird.

Using the back of the spoon, Jaypal spread the salve over a silver-dollar-sized circle around the fontanelle. Then he took a large green leaf — betel, I would later learn — and placed it on top of the goop, which glued the leaf to the skull. He wrapped a piece of cotton cloth around my chin to the crown of my skull and tied a knot on top to secure it — to keep the leaf from moving while I slept. It looked like one of those antique illustrations of someone with a toothache. When I woke up, the bandage was still in place.

This medicine, Krishna would later tell me, takes 108 days to make. The first day milk is added to the herbs, and then boiled off. Each subsequent day, more milk is added and it's boiled again, the butterfat cooking into the herbs. How the ancients figured out such elaborate methods of preparation, nobody knows.

I'd been favorably impressed with what Chandukutty had done in the 14 days I'd spent with him the year before. Still, it never occurred to me that this medicine was actually going to bring back my soft spot. That part of my skull had felt completely ossified. I guess I had retained some of my doctorly skepticism. I also knew that hyperbole is common in India, even from someone like Chandukutty who doesn't need to exaggerate. And hyperbole is common in ancient yogic texts, too, which promise that certain practices can cure any disease.

So after I bathed and removed the medicine from my head, I never checked the fontanelle. That night Jaypal returned to put on the medicine again. The following afternoon, I probed that area of the skull with my finger. *Are you kidding me?* I thought. *It worked!* There was soft indentation that hadn't been there before. Twelve years later, it's still soft.

———————

I lie face-down on Ginny Jurken's massage table, my head resting in a cradle attached to one end. She's a physical therapist, bodyworker, and yoga therapist, and is both a friend and a colleague. We are in her light-filled office in suburban Milwaukee, not far from where my sister Debbie lives. Our house growing up was inside the city limits, though I left at 19 for college in Madison and haven't lived here since.

It's four months after finishing chemoradiation, and I am here to teach a workshop at Ginny's yoga studio. But the main reason we scheduled this trip was so that she could give me a series of treatments with myofascial release (MFR). This bodywork modality was developed by another physical therapist named John Barnes. What differentiates MFR from many other styles of therapeutic massage and bodywork is that it directs its therapeutic attention to blockages and restrictions in the fascia.

Ginny is digging her elbow into the rope-like muscles that run along either side of the spine just beneath the surface. She presses down and moves very slowly, inch by painful inch, over the course of several minutes. "Aw-wwwwwwww. You're killing me!!!" I say. I don't know what the proverbial ice pick in my back would actually feel like, but this is my first guess. Since I never utter the word "Stop," this is not going to deter Ginny. I do my deepest Darth-Vader-on-a-Stairmaster breath, trying to get through it.

She's employing a myofascial release technique called soft-tissue mobilization, which is used in particularly stuck areas. She starts on my upper back on the right side, directly over where I have two healed vertebral compression fractures. These bones, the 6th and 7th of the thoracic spine, as well as several other vertebrae, are fused together. So are the joints between the spine and various ribs. All of this was caused by the fall from the second story window that happened when I was a kid.

Looking back at old photos, including one taken on the beach in Florida, I can see from the way my upper back is arching that the bones had not yet fused. I suspect that didn't happen until some time in my early 20s — forming a natural splint to protect the spinal cord. Every day in my yoga practice, I try to mobilize these vertebrae. I had assumed that it was the bones that were preventing further opening. Ginny apparently disagrees. She finds another zinger and once again I say, "You're killing me!"

———————

Fascia consists of fibrous particles of the protein collagen suspended in a gelatinous fluid known as ground substance. The watery tissue is translucent and silvery, and gives ligaments and tendon their sheen. Collagen is by weight stronger than the steel in skyscrapers due to a sturdy braid-like triple helix alignment of fibers. Fascia is able to transmit tensile forces throughout the body but also has elastic properties due to a smaller amount of another fiber, elastin.

Fascia is a living, dynamic tissue, not inert packing material as had been assumed by generations of doctors and anatomists. The orientation of its fibers changes based on how we use our bodies. Areas under constant or repeated use get thicker, with fibers aligning themselves to offer greater support. If an area is unused due to a sedentary lifestyle or sometimes due to scarring, the fibers may be laid down in a disorganized fashion, losing springiness and resiliency. Fibroblasts, cells interspersed in the connective tissue matrix, produce the fibers and direct the near-constant remodeling, yet make up less than five percent of fascia's volume. This connective tissue network envelops every muscle, and every part of every muscle: the blood vessels, the bones, and the organs. It forms one dense interpenetrating web throughout the entire body, right down to the cellular level.

I learned almost nothing about fascia in medical school, and it continues to be mostly ignored in physician education. Although doctors talk about muscles, tendons (which link muscles and bones), and ligaments (which link bones to other bones) as if they were separate entities, they are not. When you look at them under a microscope, there is no clear dividing line where muscle becomes tendon and tendon becomes bone. All of these structures blend into each other, with cells in the transition zones possessing

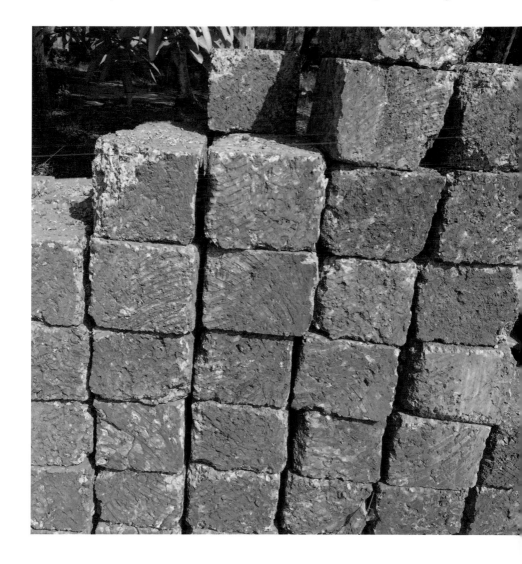

characteristics of both. They are all parts of one unified whole, which is referred to as the myofascia.

Even though doctors observe fascia when they do human dissections as medical students, they rarely think about it in the day-to-day practice of medicine. What doctors learn in medical school is what you might call "static" anatomy, based on cadaver dissections. I think this is why Dr. Morrison, the ENT surgeon down south, couldn't understand from an anatomical standpoint how tugging on my ear could open my Eustachian tubes. He was probably thinking about the muscles but not the connective tissue that binds them together. In reality, muscles don't act alone. They coordinate their actions like the members of a symphony orchestra.

The fascia surrounding any particular muscle is part of one continuous web throughout the body. Every part is connected to every other. Even muscles that supposedly exert opposing forces — one flexing and the other extending a joint, for example — affect each other via the fascia. If you tug on one part of a sweater you are wearing, a chain of tensional forces visibly affects distant areas of the garment. So too with the fascia.

Rather than learning just static anatomy, yogis and bodyworkers study the body as it lives, breathes, and moves. Their embodied understanding of anatomy is based on function, and they look at patterns of interconnection. Both approaches to anatomy have their uses. It's helpful to think, as doctors do, about individual muscles. But to view them in isolation has its limits. Reductionism strikes again. Healers like Ginny have studied reductionist anatomy in detail, but their view of the body is utterly holistic.

Ginny has been teaching health professional students in Marquette University's gross anatomy lab for two decades. After practicing physical therapy for years, she changed her practice to strictly MFR. Why? Because she found MFR so much more effective in her own healing and for her patients than conventional PT techniques. Several skeptical professors from the local medical school, who'd heard of her through colleagues, have come to her as a last resort. They wound up as regulars, persuaded by their experiences, even if they couldn't explain medically how it worked.

My treatments with Ginny are part of my ongoing efforts to prevent fibrosis in my neck — the dreaded late-appearing aftereffect of chemoradiation. Being a holistic modality, however, MFR improves the function of the neck by working on the entire body, not just the neck itself. People have a misconception that bodywork is like a massage that you might get at a spa to release tight muscles. Those usually feel wonderful, and you can relax and let your body sink in to the table. But as Ginny moves along my spine with her elbow, I am much closer to levitating off of it.

One of MFR's specialties is finding the places where there are restrictions in the mobility of fascia, which are often sensitive to the touch. The therapist meets such restrictions with sustained, gentle pressure. MFR practitioners develop the sensitivity in their hands to tell when restricted tissue is letting go. Then they follow the tactile trail to the next spot, perhaps a millimeter or two away, perhaps much further afield, where there is holding.

The post-traumatic fusing of the bones in my spine — ankylosing, as it's known medically — has rendered my backbone as hard as cement. It has amazed any number of bodyworkers who've laid their hands on it over the years, though no conventional MD has ever noticed anything out of the ordinary. "Spines like yours," Krishna told me the first time I arrived at Chandukutty Vaidyar's clinic in Kerala, "we are not seeing."

Next Ginny probes the right side of my neck, just above the collarbone. This is where the sternocleidomastoid (SCM) muscle connects the skull behind the ear to the collar bone. It's also where my cancerous lymph nodes were. On this first day that Ginny works on me, she feels a thickness in the tissue around the SCM that she concludes is a scar from the chemoradiation. I've always had difficulty turning my head, especially to the right. But the scarring in the tissue has locked it down further.

When Ginny is finished, I feel washed out but good. Also loose. She watches as I get up from the table and come into a yoga pose. I choose a simple standing back bend known as Warrior 1, the leg out in front bending at the knee. My arms are held like a Saguaro cactus as I inhale. In my most stuck area, exactly where Ginny had been trying to assassinate me, I can feel increased ease and new movement.

The bones are still fused and will remain so but I can feel that something is releasing. Since it can't be the bones, I suspect it's the myofascia that surrounds those bones. And due to myofascial connections, the greater freedom I discover in my back is allowing more movement in the neck as well. When one released area helps open another, Ginny calls it "the voice of the fascia."

———————

Over the next couple of days, Ginny works the stuck area in my neck and neighboring tissues. There are a few myofascial release techniques that she wants to do that involve going deep into the SCM muscles to reach the soft tissue in front of the cervical spine, but she can't do them because the muscles on each side of my neck do not budge. Even so, what is striking is that at the end of the second day when we test the range-of-motion (ROM) in my neck, I can turn my head to the right two inches farther than before we'd started. Even before the radiation therapy, I'd never come close to doing that.

I have a scoliosis as well, likely also a result of the childhood accident — my thoracic spine and rib cage rotate to the right. When we view my body at the end of the second day in front of her full-length mirror, the symmetry in my spine, head and neck has improved. We shoot a photo and regret not having taken one the day before. In the past, with therapeutic massage and some other bodywork techniques, I experienced some opening of stuck tissues on the table, but within a day or two, I would be back to where I started. What's surprising me about MFR is that the changes seem to persist. In the months after Ginny added two inches to my neck turning, I wouldn't lose any of it.

Four months after finishing chemoradiation, my left ear had finally cleared, but when I arrived in Milwaukee to work with Ginny, my right ear was still blocked. One day, I am lying on my back and Ginny decides to work on my right calf. As she pulls the leg toward where she stands at the foot of the table, my right ear pops. Immediately my hearing normalizes, but the effect only lasts a minute. Later, she does the same pull and the Eustachian tube opens again.

Two day later, Ginny is again working on my right leg. The blocked ear opens once more, and this time it stays clear. That tugging on my calf would help my Eustachian tube to open seems even crazier than the notion that pulling on the ear would, but the fascia around the

Eustachian tubes is connected to both. It wasn't her intention, but by working on my legs, Ginny had elicited the fascial voice in a far-flung area of the body.

And lo and behold, I could hear it.

―――――――――――

Most days Ginny complements the hands-on work she does with passive stretches of fascia. I lie over some combination of foam rollers and balls of various sizes and consistencies. She might have me lie on the table in her treatment room in something like a supported Corpse pose, Shavasana, with a three-inch diameter squishy plastic ball just under my tail bone. Then she'll place a slightly larger and firmer ball under a tight muscle in my left lower back that connects the ribs to the pelvic rim. She often sticks a foam roller under my Achilles tendons at the back of both ankles. Lying on these props I'm using my own body weight to provide gentle, sustained pressure. Areas of the fascia she can't reach — which chain to the areas she's working on — get released. When they release, the fascia beneath her fingers lets go more readily.

Today Ginny places a hand-made wooden roller under my back. It's four inches long, and is carved out in the middle and raised on both sides. The bumps dig into the muscles on both sides of my spine simultaneously, just where she'd worked so painfully with her elbow. I hold the position for a few minutes, and when she wants to target another area, she moves the wood implement up or down the spine.

Under my neck is a smaller, firm foam roller. To encourage the opening of the tissues there, she has me turn my head just far enough to the side that the SCM muscle attaching behind the ear is compressed. This elicits the dull, burning sensation that I've come to associate with fascial opening. It's uncomfortable, but I know it's doing me good.

Ginny lends me a few balls and rollers to take back to my room at Debbie's house. My assignment is to spend time on them every day, making my MFR intensive all the more so.

———————

Staying at Debbie's place during my MFR treatments is easy. She lets me use her car to get to my appointments with Ginny, even if it means someone else will need to pick her up from her job at the hardware store. Debbie had even offered to let me stay at their place during my cancer treatment if I had wanted to get treated at a medical center near them. Although my sister and I don't get to see each other much, we've maintained a sweet relationship over the years, so it's good to get this chance to be together now. Her husband John, a lawyer who works for a non-profit and whose company I've always enjoyed, catches me up on the crazy ups and down of Wisconsin politics as we stroll around the neighborhood some evenings.

———————

Most people — and most doctors — are unaware that if you slouch all the time, you may lose your ability to sit and stand up straight. If you don't use a part of your body, the fascia in that area tends to contract, making it almost impossible to stretch that area. Over time, the fascia and the muscles it envelops keep shortening, locking you into the poor posture that started out as only a bad habit.

That is exactly what happened to me. When I started practicing yoga, I'd been rounding my back into a C-shaped slump for decades. I carried my head several inches in front of my spine. In that position, the SCM muscles were never stretched and over time they became significantly shorter. The same thing happened to the pectoralis minor, a short muscle that connects the front of the shoulder blade to three of the upper ribs. All of this reinforced my lousy posture.

When I first started to practice asana with Patricia in Cambridge, any back-bending poses were nearly impossible. The fusion in my spine hadn't been diagnosed yet, but clearly, it was limiting me. With years of yoga practice, though, and hundreds of sessions of bodywork — most recently MFR — I continue to gain new opening. This is happening even at a time of life when most people are steadily losing range of motion.

Nearly every holistic modality I've been using lacks the scientific support that evidence-based medicine demands. If I consider myself a scientist, and I do, why didn't I let this lack of evidence dissuade me? Let me explain.

Research that follows the dictates of EBM can be an excellent tool to evaluate reductionist therapies. It's also valuable when comparing one reductionist approach to another. It was scientific evidence that led me to choose low-dose, weekly Cisplatin chemotherapy over the higher-dose, intermittent protocol. And I chose to reject the proposed radical neck surgery because there was no evidence the operation was any more effective than chemoradiation.

When it comes to evaluating holistic approaches, I believe that EBM — at least as it is currently practiced — is the wrong tool for the job. EBM was created by reductionists to evaluate reductionist treatments. But trying to shove the round peg of holism into that square hole is unfair. It makes holistic treatments look ineffective even when they work.

Medical research is expensive. Most research these days is funded by industry — but there are no deep pockets to fund research into holistic remedies. Why no deep pockets? Because holistic approaches can't be patented — no patents means no monopolies on production, and no big profits. Holistic researchers rely instead on either government or foundations, but these won't fund studies that don't follow EBM's rules. If holistic researchers don't play the EBM game, their research does not get done. If they do play the game, and shoehorn holistic treatments into reductionist research protocols, the results are likely to be biased.

Some holistic tools, say a mantra or a low dose of an herb, might not be powerful enough to generate a statistically significant difference in a disease process when studied in isolation. But when working synergistically as part of a holistic regimen, they might indeed contribute to overall effectiveness. EBM insists on studying each element of a treatment approach one at a time, so such research does not detect synergetic benefits — yet can be used as evidence that the treatments are ineffective.

Worse, due to funding problems most holistic remedies never get studied at all. What manufacturer will fund a study of an herb that any competitor could sell? Who's going to pay for studies of fasting? It wasn't that the holistic modalities I was considering during my cancer care had been shown to be ineffective — most hadn't ever been studied.

On top of that, EBM demands that there be experimental evidence of the effectiveness of a treatment *for each and every medical condition* it's used for. That means not just for cancer, but for each of the more than 100 types of cancer. No exception is made for holistic treatments. But this demand misses what holistic healing is all about.

Yoga therapists like to say that they treat people, not conditions. Holistic treatments don't attack diseases per se; they strengthen and balance the person to better fight any disease.

Most reductionist treatments are only aimed at one or a few conditions, so the insistence on disease-by-disease proof doesn't present a huge obstacle. Holistic healing, on the other hand, could be useful in any medical condition. To study each of the many diseases a holistic modality like yoga could treat would be astronomically expensive. This requirement alone ensures that most holistic approaches will never be able to amass the amount of evidence that EBM requires. It also means that private insurers and health care systems that follow EBM's standards in deciding what they'll pay for will never approve most holistic treatments.

EBMers didn't place this burden on holistic therapies to be unfair — even though this is very much the effect. They did it because dividing up the terrain of medicine into discrete diseases is how reductionists think. But it makes no sense when applied to holistic healing. It's an example of what I call "reductionism ad absurdum."

But there's an even more insidious bias built into virtually all studies of holistic healing. To understand this bias, I need to go into more detail. Read on.

Some scientific studies have shown that holistic approaches don't work, when clinical experience indicates that they do. This disconnect is far more common than you might suppose. The problem often arises because of the way in which EBM requires studies to be conducted.

A case in point: You may have seen the headlines some years ago proclaiming, "Acupuncture No More Effective than Sham Treatment." These were prompted by a study in a prominent medical journal of people with migraine headaches. At the beginning of the trial, the patients averaged more than five days per month debilitated by migraines of moderate to severe intensity. After the treatment, the number of headache days decreased by about half for both the acupuncture and the sham treatment. The people on the waiting list, who later received acupuncture treatment, improved much less.

The results were taken as evidence that acupuncture only works via the placebo effect. Acupuncture skeptics jumped all over the findings. Why would anyone in his or her right mind use this nonsensical treatment?

The study was a randomized, placebo-controlled trial — which EBM considers the gold standard of proof. The participants who received "real" acupuncture were needled at acupoints considered helpful for migraines. The participants who received "sham" acupuncture were needled only superficially, and at non-acupoints.

Both the real acupuncture and the sham version were delivered by medical acupuncturists. These were physicians who had been trained in Chinese medicine for at least 140 hours. Many of the articles I read in popular magazines when I began seriously investigating holistic healing in the mid-1990s recommended these MDs over traditionally-trained acupuncturists. These doctors learn to choose points based on the western medical diagnosis and were presumably viewed as more scientific.

Traditional practitioners of Chinese medicine in the West do not study for a hundred-something hours. Their training programs run for *thousands* of hours, typically over a three-year period. A healer like Hiroyuki would have logged tens of thousands of hours of training, starting in early childhood.

More importantly, traditional practitioners learn an entire diagnostic system that medical acupuncturists do not — and that system is crucial to selecting the correct points to needle. What western medicine sees as a single diagnosis, migraine headache, would be seen in Chinese medicine as arising from any of a great number of imbalances. Any of these could cause a migraine, and the TCM acupuncturist assesses which patterns each individual has — and chooses the treatments accordingly.

The TCM practitioner assesses the patient by taking a complete history, as well as by examination of the patient's pulse, tongue, and as we saw with Hiroyuki, abdomen. Although traditional acupuncturists rely on observable phenomena, it can take years to master these diagnostic techniques, and skills grow with steady use over long periods of time. Practitioners might choose a variety of treatment approaches including herbs, moxibustion and acupuncture, each one designed to address some aspect of the patient's disharmony, as determined by such an examination. They might also offer personalized dietary and lifestyle advice. A treatment aimed at one pattern of disharmony could be inappropriate, and even harmful for another one.

In TCM, there is no one-size-fits-all fix for migraine headaches. Any studies of a system like traditional acupuncture that insist on using a standardized treatment protocol based on the western medical diagnosis will underestimate the value of the approach. Inevitably, some subjects, and probably many, in any treatment-by-diagnosis study will be getting the incorrect treatment, as understood in Chinese medicine.

Needling acupuncture points that are chosen according to a western medical diagnosis is a reductionist version of a deep holistic system. There may be some benefit

— but even at its best, it's a pale imitation of TCM. Did this study show that "real" acupuncture is no more effective than "sham" acupuncture? Or did it show that one type of sham acupuncture was no more effective than another type of sham acupuncture? Maybe the proper conclusion to draw is that a watered-down version of holistic acupuncture was not good enough to be found significantly better statistically than a placebo. The real sham was the testing protocol.

No serious side effects developed in response to either real or fake needling in the acupuncture study. No patients withdrew due to side effects — something rarely seen in drug studies. Indeed, in the hands of a well-trained acupuncturist who uses sterilized needles, the treatment is safer than virtually anything in conventional medicine. One huge study in Japan found that side effects occurred in one of every 5,000 patients. These adverse effects included bruising (often painless), redness, or pain at puncture sites. The most serious one was a fall from bed.

The authors of the sham acupuncture study attributed whatever good came of the acupuncture, real and sham, to the placebo effect. Evidence-based medicine is obsessed in its research with ruling out any therapeutic benefits that could be attributed to placebo. Dr. Hamblin gave alternate nostril breathing the ultimate EBM kiss-off: It's nothing more than a placebo. It's as if they believe the placebo effect is a bad thing. It's not.

The placebo response can be a powerful tool that influences the actual effectiveness of *any* treatment — from surgery to prescription drugs to chanting mantra. Studies consistently have found placebo helps roughly one third of people, almost regardless of diagnosis. Placebo has been shown in studies to be as effective as arthroscopic surgery in mitigating knee pain. Placebo induces remissions from clinical depression as well as antidepressant drugs. Closer to home for me, placebo can bolster the effectiveness of chemotherapy. Indeed, placebo is so good that doctors ought to be doing everything they can to facilitate it in every clinical encounter. This is what Dr. Clark did for me with the simple gesture of putting his hand on my shoulder, and calling me "brother." I felt better immediately.

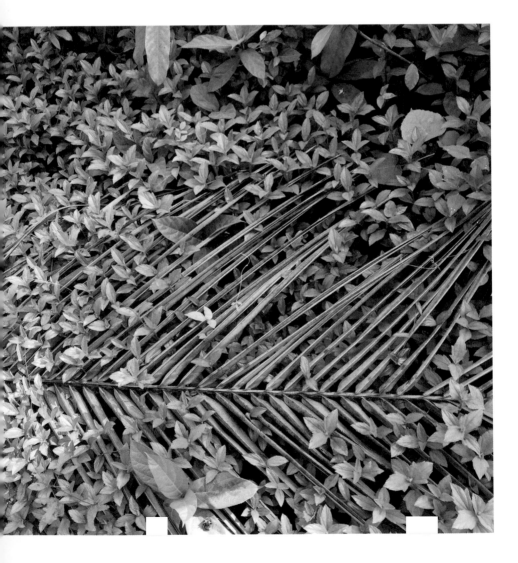

Physicians no doubt mean well when they reject alternative therapies — after all, they're not supported by evidence. They do this even when those treatments pose little or no risk. There's no evidence, it's unscientific! they proclaim — using EBM's narrow definition of what constitutes evidence. You have to wonder if doctors knew that their words had such power, would they so cavalierly dismiss treatments that might benefit patients, even if only from placebo? Patients look up to doctors. When a physician dismisses a treatment, patients naturally expect less and their symptoms may worsen. This is placebo's evil twin — "the nocebo effect," as medicine calls it.

It's beyond me why any physician wouldn't want to make use of such a powerful tool — one that doesn't cost a penny. Good healers — holistic and conventional — make their patients feel cared for. This alone may be enough to heal some ills. This is the placebo effect skillfully employed. But in the rushed world of conventional healthcare, there isn't as much room for human interaction as there used to be. Holistic healers spend much more time with their patients, which may help them evoke a greater placebo response.

Hiroyuki had been trained in acupuncture since childhood. He didn't normally use it in Massachusetts, though — he wasn't licensed by the State to practice it. Even without needles, he could almost always use other tools to get the desired results. The only exception was when I'd developed a viral meningitis in the year 2000 that sent me to the emergency room. He had seen me a few days earlier. When I called him to describe my illness, he got mad at himself. He believed that he should have seen the warning signs — and prevented the meningitis from ever happening.

That prompted Hiroyuki to bring me in for a special session. When I arrived, he brought out a wood case about the size of a toolbox. Inside were acupuncture needles of many sizes, and made from different materials. There were wooden ones as big as knitting needles, designed to stimulate acupoints on the skin but not penetrate it.

This was the only time I got to experience Hiroyuki's acupuncture. It was a virtuoso performance like nothing I've witnessed before or since. Holding a needle, he uncapped it with the same hand, while his other arm moved in a balletic gesture of counterbalance. Every movement appeared choreographed like a classical Indian dancer's. Chandukutty Vaidyar is the only other holistic healer in whom I've witnessed this level of mastery.

From the small sample I saw, I imagined Hiroyuki was likely to be the best acupuncturist in the state. I had seen his general level of mastery without needles. I knew he was on the faculty at the big acupuncture college in the area, yet the Commonwealth of Massachusetts did not allow him to practice the art of acupuncture. Although his spoken English was fluent, I'd heard he'd failed the written exam and had been unwilling to retake it.

He got around the state's restriction on practicing acupuncture that day by refusing to accept any payment for the appointment.

———

Masters of ancient healing systems like Hiroyuki and my teacher Chandukutty Vaidyar typically begin their studies in childhood. They were guided by masters, often their fathers and grandfathers, who in turn learned from theirs. In my experience, these are the real virtuosos of the field. A child who starts playing the violin or tennis at the age of four can achieve a level of accomplishment impossible for anyone who takes it up as an adult. These masters are head-and-shoulders above anyone who trained only after college, even if these people get a fabulous education.

If we really want to assess whether ancient healing systems like Ayurveda and TCM are effective, I believe we ought to be studying the work of such masters. This might allow us to establish once and for all that modalities like Ayurveda and traditional Asian medicine are effective, even if the explanations for how they work don't make sense to most western scientists.

EBM assumes that a careful study of a reductionist imitation of a real holistic treatment (as we saw in the sham acupuncture study) is superior to a muddier statistical look at the real thing — but there is not one iota of scientific evidence to support this belief. We could test that idea by comparing the effectiveness of a standardized protocol to the work of a master. It would have to be an outcomes study — the masters must be allowed to do what they do unfettered, using whatever combination of tools they judge best. They must also be allowed to change the protocol as needed along the way, based on their observations of the patient's state. That's what good practitioners always do.

Outcomes studies simply assess whether a group benefitted from treatments compared to a control group. They don't require the treatments to be standardized. Reductionists want to be able to isolate the "active ingredient," and outcomes studies don't let you do that. But that's a reductionist notion — it doesn't apply that much to holistic healing.

As far as I know, studies comparing masterfully tailored treatments to one-size-fits-all protocols have never been done. What if the personalized approach turned out to be superior — as I believe is nearly certain? It would undermine the whole philosophical underpinning of the way EBM insists holistic healing must be studied. Maybe that's why the experiment never gets done.

———————

One western scientist who has made serious inquiries into the effectiveness of acupuncture is Harvard Medical School's Helene Langevin, MD. Dr. Langevin got interested in it almost by accident. Working as an endocrinologist, she had patients in chronic pain who inquired about acupuncture. She was skeptical, but also frustrated by the lack of effectiveness of the usual treatment options: pain relievers and conventional physical therapy. She decided to investigate acupuncture by enrolling in a local hands-on course, she wrote, "if only to be able to respond to patient questions more intelligently."

She was taught to twirl the acupuncture needles until she felt resistance like the tug on a line when a fish bites the hook. She could feel it, and got curious about what was happening anatomically. Her instructor told her it was from muscles contracting around the needle. She knew it couldn't be that, because she could feel it in areas like the wrist where there are no muscles under the acupoint.

Trying to understand what that tug meant led her to an interest in connective tissue and its role in chronic pain. In a study she did while at the University of Vermont, she and her colleagues looked under the microscope at animal tissue in which acupuncture needles had been twisted. They could see the connective tissue under the skin "wrap around the needle, like spaghetti winding around a fork." She realized that was what led to the tug she felt when turning the needle. And since the fascia is interconnected, this results in a stretching of the neighboring fascia.

These forces, she wrote, can be transmitted all the way to the interior of cells, and result in the release of signaling molecules or changes in gene expression.

Most of us learned in biology class that cells are like fluid-filled bags, in which mitochondria and other organelles float. It turns out that there is a connective tissue lattice, a "cytoskeleton," inside every cell to which organelles are attached. The cytoskeleton is even linked to the nucleus which houses the cell's DNA, where genes may be switched on or off. Crucial in linking the outside and inside of cells are proteins called integrins, which span the cell membrane. Integrins connect to the fascia on the outside and to the cytoskeleton on the inside.

When connective tissues get stuck together from trauma, scarring, or due to chronic inflammation or poor postural habits, movement is restricted. Cancer cells have been shown to spread more easily in such places. Thus, in theory, yoga, acupuncture, and bodywork like MFR, by helping to relieve such fascial restrictions, could make the tissues less receptive to cancer invasion and spread. One of the studies that Dr. Langevin and other Harvard researchers did to research this possibility involved mice.

At the start of the study, the mice were injected with breast cancer cells in the fat pads near the breast. Then the researchers suspended the animals by their tails, allowing them to grasp a bar with their front paws, stretching their entire torsos. The mice could comfortably hold this position for 10 minutes. With their tiny spines angled down, they were stretched once a day in a pose that might be called Downward-Facing Mouse. The other mice, the control group, weren't stretched.

The experiment ran for four weeks. The tumor growth of the stretched mice was significantly slower from weeks two to four than the tumor growth in the non-stretched controls. By the end of the study, the mice that had stretched the subcutaneous connective tissue of their torsos and front legs had tumors that were 52 percent smaller than the control group's.

———————

My oncologists had no idea why my cancer spread to the lymph nodes on the opposite side of my neck and not the ones on the same side — but I think I know. For years, I've noticed that when I practice asana the prana on the right side of my body is partially blocked. I can feel the difference between the two sides. The line of dysfunction extends from the right side of my chest up to the right side of the neck. It also runs through the right abdomen, all the way down to my right foot. All of this, I believe, is the aftereffect on my bones and fascia of a couple of serious childhood injuries. But I figured that my doctors wouldn't know what to make of my theory, so I decided to not mention it.

———————

With my medical background, I was steeped in the "medical model," the notion that treatments should be based on the diagnosis. When I got interested in yoga therapy, I assumed the same idea would apply. What I read encouraged this belief. BKS Iyengar, the yoga master whom I was fortunate enough to spend time with before he died, wrote the best-selling yoga book of all time, *Light on Yoga*. In the back, he recommended specific yoga poses and sequences of poses based upon western medical diagnoses.

As I observed his therapeutic work in the "medical classes" at his Institute in Pune, it soon became obvious that he didn't use the routines he'd recommended in that or any of his other books. Instead, based on each student's particular situation, Iyengar developed a sequence just for them. And, as I learned, as the student's condition changed in response to the yoga he prescribed or other developments, Iyengar continually tweaked the practice.

Often, I watched him call out the name of a pose he wanted a student to be put in. His assistants would scramble to set up the bolsters and other props and get the student into position. But, not infrequently, as soon as Iyengar saw the result, he'd wave his arms and say, "Take her out."

Based on something he saw, he knew the pose wouldn't serve the student. Perhaps her breath had become rough. Maybe he didn't like the way her spine looked. He didn't say.

Iyengar was arguably one of the best yoga therapists in the world, if not the best. Yet he couldn't anticipate, even with a student he knew well, if a particular pose was going to work until he saw the student do it. If that's the case, I wondered, how can any canned yoga sequence, or any "standardized protocol" used in a study — designed by someone who has never laid eyes on the patients who will do it — accurately capture what good yoga therapists actually do?

To get a yoga study funded by either the government or foundations, you need to follow the rules of EBM. As with one-size-fits-all acupuncture, researchers must employ a fixed set of yoga postures or other techniques that everyone in the experimental group does. If everyone doesn't do exactly the same regimen, then the study would be considered methodologically weak, and funding would not be approved.

In other words, researchers are only allowed to study "dumbed-down," reductionist versions of yoga therapy. Most yoga researchers know that this requirement is problematic, since that's not how the best therapists practice. If you want to do research, though, you've got to play by rules — ill-advised as they may be. These canned sequences will not be optimal for many, or most, of the patients studied. For some, they could be counterproductive. Once again, following the letter of EBM's law means that study results will consistently underestimate yoga's powers.

———————————

There has been a huge growth in integrative medicine in hospitals and clinics in the United States. There are journals and conferences dedicated to promoting its scientific basis, and there has been a big push to make the field more "evidence-based." On one level this is fantastic. But there's a problem. The overwhelming majority of the research in complementary and alternative medicine (CAM) is of alternative reductionist therapies, not of holistic approaches.

Reductionist treatments like drugs, megadose vitamins and dietary supplements lend themselves much better to placebo-controlled, randomized controlled trials (RCTs) — which, as we've discussed, is the gold standard of proof in EBM. Because of this, studies of alternative reductionist therapies are much more likely to be judged by scientists as of high methodological quality — and with industry supporting alternative reductionist research, a lot more of it gets done.

Unfortunately, holistic approaches don't fit as nicely into the preferred testing protocol. For some like yoga, there aren't even credible placebos that "real" yoga could be compared to. How do you convince someone who's not doing yoga that they're doing yoga? This means that all yoga studies are not placebo-controlled — and therefore are considered less scientifically rigorous. That is not yoga's fault, and it shouldn't be penalized for it.

Unfortunately, the more "evidence-based" an integrative physician's approach is, the more likely it's going to be dominated by alternative reductionist therapies at the expense of holistic therapies. The way I see it, if alternative medicine becomes little more than alternative reductionism, that's not much of an alternative.

———————

Recently, I read a review of the scientific evidence of yoga's effectiveness in heart disease. Practicing yoga regularly appears to improve a number of risk factors for heart attacks, such as blood pressure and blood sugar levels. Numerous studies including dozens of randomized controlled trials (RCTs) report these benefits. But to the experts, there was not enough evidence to conclude that yoga works for those at risk of or who've already suffered

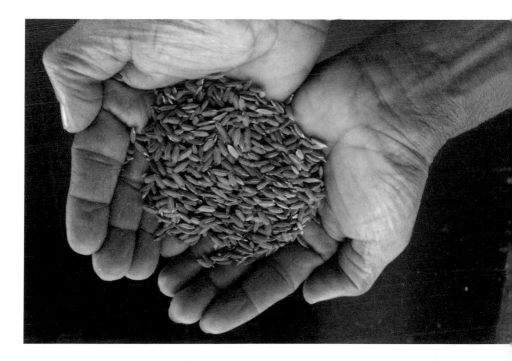

a heart attack. Nor, they concluded, was there enough data to comment on the safety of the practice.

Interestingly, the scientists doing the analysis omitted the work of Dr. Dean Ornish. The studies of his revolutionary approach to heart disease were published in top-drawer conventional medical journals, but because Ornish uses a number of modalities in his program, his studies are outcome studies, which, as explained earlier, reductionist scientists look down on.

Ornish's program combines yoga with a number of elements of traditional yogic lifestyle, like smoking cessation and a plant-based diet. He based his program on the lifestyle at the ashram of his teacher, Swami Satchidananda. Ornish included yoga, breathing, and meditation practices from the ashram but left out the Sanskrit mantras, ghee lamps, and elephant-headed deities.

Based on his research, we can conclude that a multi-faceted yoga and lifestyle intervention appears to be both safe and effective in not only arresting — but reversing — the progression of blockages in coronary arteries. His patients did much better than those in the control group whose medical care included cardiac procedures like bypass surgery and cholesterol-lowering medications. Furthermore, his program has proved to be both safe and cost-effective.

Even though EBM's methods for studying yoga are flawed, that research nonetheless is helping make the case for the practice. Most one-size-fits-all yoga protocols tested in research studies show favorable results. This helps the field gain credibility in society at large.

My impression is that even those skeptics who attack acupuncture and herbal medicine generally give yoga a pass. I believe we have the ever-growing number of published yoga studies to thank for this. Scientific research is also a huge influence on government agencies, health care professionals, and scientifically-minded members of the general public. In the case of the Ornish program, it's even led major insurance companies and the US government's Medicare program to pay for it.

Only research will persuade government and private insurers to reimburse for such treatments. Reimbursement would allow people from underserved communities, typically underrepresented in the yoga world, to gain access to these safe, effective healing tools — even if it's dumbed-down yoga. But this would fall short of the ultimate goal of researching, and broadly implementing, what the best practitioners actually do.

Research scientists, following the dictates of EBM, attempt to discern the "actual" effectiveness of a treatment, by which they mean the measured effectiveness, after they've subtracted out any part that is due to placebo. This allows doctors (or so they believe) to judge which treatments are best for patients, and to make "science-based" recommendations. But this belief is mistaken. What is best for patients is what is most effective overall, which means the combination of the therapeutic efficacy of the treatment itself *plus* anything that comes from patients' expectations, their trust in their practitioners, and the other elements that comprise the placebo effect.

If a treatment helps, patients are often less concerned than doctors and researchers with why. Patients are simply looking for relief. If part or even all of the benefit is due to the placebo effect, who cares?

Back in Vermont in the autumn months before my return to India, I am lying in my favorite restorative yoga pose: Legs up the Wall, with my pelvis supported by a bolster. I slip my index finger into my mouth, and start to do what in MFR is known as "intra-oral" work. Using the pad of the finger I press on the gum above my upper molars until I feel the resistance and ache of the connective tissue. Applying gentle pressure, I wait until I feel the tissue let go. When one area releases, I move my finger along to the area above a neighboring tooth, again probing for tightness.

The MFR technique I'm employing I learned from Ginny last summer, though it's my elaboration to do it in a restorative yoga pose. It's similar to what I've experienced in another system of bodywork, Rolfing, which also aims to treat the fascia.

Mouth work is, I believe, one of the most powerful ways I've found to try to prevent fibrosis of the neck. I'm sure I'm not as good at it as Ginny is, but I've gotten better over time and I can feel that it's making a difference. And of course, when I do it, it's free of cost, and I can do it as often as I like.

I work all around both tonsils and the root of the tongue, which had gotten so tight during my radiation treatments. Even areas that made me gag at first, I acclimated to over time. Mouth works also allows me to monitor if there's anything growing that I would need to get checked out. When I first explored the roof of my mouth with my thumb and had a deep nervous system release, it made me understand how powerful thumb sucking must be for an infant. I imagine breast feeding causes a similar reaction, though I never got to experience that as a baby.

Sometimes when I'm palpating soft tissues in my mouth, emotions like sadness come up. If so, I try to simply notice them mindfully, without judgment. After I finish a session of mouth work, which might last 10 minutes, staying in the same restorative pose, I immediately sink into a state of profound relaxation, much deeper than I'm typically able to achieve.

"Use your feeling brain, not your thinking brain," Ginny said, as her fingers sank into the tissue at the back of my neck. One of the muscles connecting the shoulder blade to the neck, I had told her, felt like a rope. She was working to soften it, and to release the fascia that surrounds every fiber of this and every muscle. I closed my eyes and focused on the sensation, encouraging the area to relax. Something must have worked, because she immediately remarked that my body seemed more responsive to her touch.

When I can get my rational mind to step aside, even for a few minutes, things happen that otherwise wouldn't. Everything seems to go more smoothly. Over the years, I've come to rely more and more on intuition. It lets me know what's good for me and what isn't, which treatments are helping me and which aren't. Rational thinking hasn't been dismissed — I rely on it every day and couldn't live without it. You might say it still has a vote, but its veto power has been revoked.

For the last 25 years, and especially in the last decade, my intuition has prompted me to take a closer look at my early life. What has made me who I am? Which of the strategies I developed as I grew up continue to serve me well, and which ones need to be jettisoned? Who do I want to be for the rest of my life?

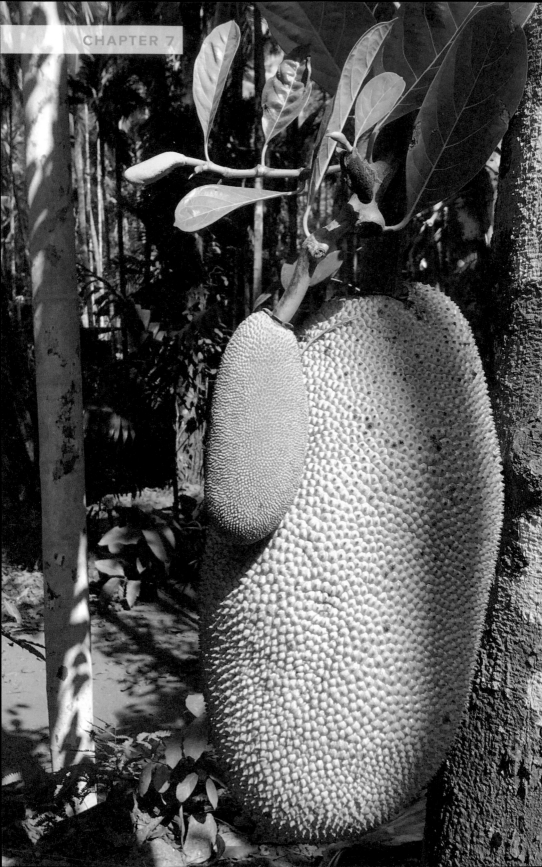

MOTHER'S LOVE

"If it had been any other surgeon," my brother Ray says, "Mom would not have survived." The renowned Dr. Davis, who was visiting the famous maternity hospital where I was born, performed the elective C-section a few weeks before the due date. Mom had been having third trimester bleeding from placenta previa, which obstructed the birth canal.

"The baby's had its chance," Dr. Davis had told her. "Now it's your turn."

The pregnancy had not been an easy one. Mom had been told that if the bleeding started again, she had six minutes to get to the hospital or she might bleed to death. It was a 14-minute drive from our house in Chicago's Hyde Park neighborhood. Hundreds of Masses were said all over the city for the two of us.

Mom was in her early 40s, old for a mother in those days. My father, who preferred to be called Pop, told me that he and Mom had tried for years to have more children. They'd had some difficulty conceiving, had lost a few babies to miscarriages and had assumed my mother was no longer fertile. That's why I sometimes call myself a "menopause surprise." But when it came down to it, as my older brother Ray tells me, she wasn't happy being pregnant so late in life. The complications, and her fear for her life, made her suffering all the worse.

According to Mom, "Fabulous!" is what Dr. Davis exclaimed as he opened her up. He was thrilled to be able to show such a great case to the obstetric residents gathered around the operating table. The placenta was malformed and I was so tangled up in it, Ray says, that there was almost no way to get me out. Mom was awake but nauseated during the entire delivery. Dr. Davis had told her that if she threw up, she wouldn't survive. Somehow, she managed not to vomit. As soon as I was delivered, she went for an emergency hysterectomy. I was meanwhile whisked to an incubator, an appliance about the size of a microwave oven, where I would spend most of the next month.

When I was around three, I was in love with a black cat with white paws and a patch of white on his neck, named Spats. "Spaaaaaaaaats. Psssssssbbbbbbsssssssssss-bbbbb," I'd call from my bedroom, making the sibilant sound that was our signal, and he would run in the door and nuzzle up to me.

"He comes to you like a puppy," Pop said. "Cats don't usually do that." In my baby book, Pop wrote that I didn't seem much interested in the family dog, an Irish Setter named Rusty, though I have fond memories of many of the dogs we had after that. But for several crucial years early in my life, Spats was my pal, lavishing affection on me, as I did with him.

"Pop was obsessed with you for four years," Ray says, and that's exactly how long he wrote entries in *Our Baby's First Seven Years Record Book*, which he'd bought at the hospital after I was born. "He was thrilled that he had another boy that late in life," Ray says. "He was over the moon." Pop called me his "last hostage to fortune," and I think I liked hearing that, though I had no idea what it meant.

When I went through the lake house in Vermont, sorting through our family possessions before the sale of the house became final, the tennis trophy wasn't the only meaningful personal artifact I found. But there was one treasure I'd missed. A few days after the sale went through, the buyer, God bless her, mailed me that baby book. I had never seen it before, and didn't even know it existed. Paging through it later, I would find a number of clues as to what my early days must have been like.

––––––––––

In my baby book — which Pop updated regularly in careful handwriting much different from his usual illegible scrawl — he wrote that I would burst into laughter any time Ray came into the room. This started when I was five months old. Pop wrote that Tony, who was nine when I was born, always seemed to see me as the competition. Ray, who was 12, never did. He played the role of my ally and protector.

When I was four years old, Mom and Pop bought me my first bike for Christmas. The next summer, I still couldn't ride it without training wheels. I had turned five and I knew that by then I was supposed to be able to do without them. That's when Ray stepped in. He unbolted the training wheels, and held the bike steady, while I climbed on. As I began to pedal, he relaxed his hands, but when the bike rocked side to side and I got scared, he tightened his grip. I climbed off the bike, and was reluctant to get back on. It was too unsteady.

The bike's not unsteady, he said. "It's you. Watch."

Holding the handlebars with his left hand, he placed his right behind the seat and gave it a shove. The riderless bike sailed straight and true down the sidewalk, past the house next door, all the way to the corner, where it hit the curb and folded itself to the ground.

Avuncular as he was, Ray and I still butted heads from time to time. When I was maybe six, I was watching TV sitting on everyone's favorite chair, the metal stool from the kitchen. I went to the bathroom during a commercial and while I was gone, Ray had taken possession of the stool. When I complained, he scoffed. It was his now. I sat on the sofa behind him, ticked off.

A few minutes later, Ray stood and took one long step toward the black-and-white set. He adjusted the dial, and without taking his eyes off the screen, backed up to sit down. As his skinny butt descended toward the top of the stool, I grabbed it with both hands and yanked it toward me. He hit the Oriental rug, and then the roof, two examples of instant karma. He chased me into the next room where my mother sat reading in her armchair and, for one of the only times I can remember, I jumped to her side for protection.

My parents started taking in foster children shortly after I was born. The first foster child was Pat, our teenaged paperboy, who lived in an unstable family. When he was going to be removed from his home by the authorities, a few families volunteered to take him in. In the end, he chose us because of Ray, who he'd been hanging out with for the last year. My sister Debbie, who came to live with us as a foster kid when she was three, was one year younger than I. She was the second of a dozen or so foster kids my parents took in over the years, and the only one they adopted.

Once Catholic Services, which handled foster kids, realized my mother's proclivity, they called her every now and again hoping she might take another child, which she often did. The third one was Debbie's older brother Michael, who proved more difficult to integrate into the family. If any other child got attention in his presence, he'd completely melt down.

One summer in Vermont, when I'd just turned six, we were staying at my grandparents' farmhouse, on land that adjoined the lake house property. Michael and I were fighting, and wrestling on the squishy double bed in the bedroom everyone called Grand Central. My New Yorker grandparents gave it that name because anyone sleeping in either of the other bedrooms had to pass through it to get downstairs to the only bathroom.

A year older than I, and bigger and stronger, Michael knelt over me and pinned me down. He pushed a pillow into my face and held it there. I couldn't breathe. I knew this was bad. Somehow, I managed to turn my head to one side and squirm out of harm's way. I'm not sure I ever mentioned it to my parents.

At the end of that summer, just before I was to start first grade and Michael second, my parents decided that they needed to return him to the foster agency. He was too disruptive, too hard to control. He wasn't the last foster kid they took in and then sent back. I asked Debbie recently about her reaction to Michael's departure, but she says she has no memory of it, or even of him living with us at all.

My first grade teacher, who I'll call Sister Mary Joseph, seemed to have it in for me from the get go. She was tall and scary in her floor-length black habit. Her starch-stiffened headwear made her look like the monster I knew her to be. She yelled at me, slapped me, and made fun of me in front of the class.

Early in the school year, Pop was clipping my fingernails. "Don't cut them too short," I said. I thought I might need them to scratch Sister Mary Joseph. My parents were disturbed. Pop phoned her at the convent, though he didn't tell me. The following day, she pulled me out of class and marched me to the middle of the empty auditorium, the same room where the whole school had watched the movie Pollyanna. She unfolded two metal chairs, and placed them facing each other, in the middle of the hardwood floor. She sat in one, and directed me to sit in the other, inches away. The big, bad nun then removed her rimless, stop-sign bifocals, the better to glare at me. For a long while, she said nothing.

"I understand you want to grow your fingernails out, so you can scratch me," she said.

How could she know? *God must have told her*.

Years later, Ray told me that Sister Mary Joseph had loved Michael. She'd taken him on as her personal project the year he'd spent in her classroom. She'd even asked, after years of teaching the first grade, to be transferred to the second grade, so that she could continue to teach him. Maybe she thought I was to blame for Michael's being sent away. If so, she couldn't have been too pleased to see me the first day of school.

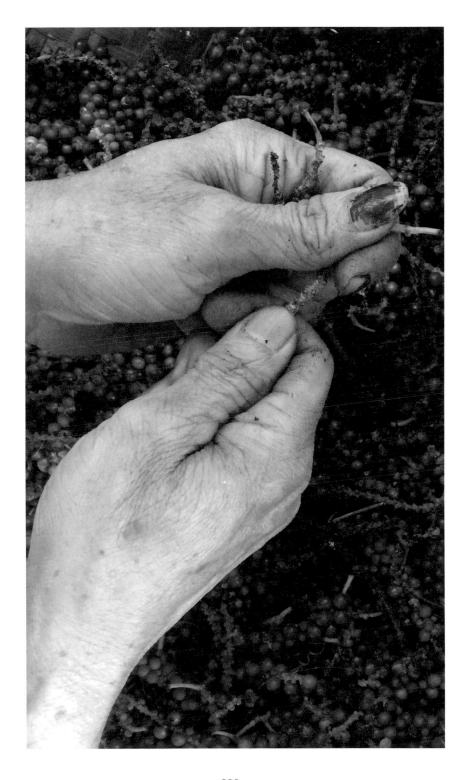

At ten, I hung around with kids who were what they used to call "juvenile delinquents," or on the road to it. And my mom, who was a better judge of character than my psychologist father, didn't like any of them. My pals and I had discovered an unlocked window in an abandoned garage near where we lived on Milwaukee's east side. The building had two floors and a dumbwaiter connecting them, and upstairs a bulbous old-fashioned car like none of us had ever seen.

Sitting upstairs, in a small window-lined room, I flicked the flint wheel on the chrome Zippo lighter that I'd shoplifted to fire up our similarly pilfered Winstons. I loved the sweet smell of the fluid. Heavy in my hand, the Zippo made a satisfying hollow click when I snapped it open, one-handed with my thumb, and closed it with my index finger, which I did repeatedly, even when nobody needed a light.

As we pulled on our cigarettes, we leafed through Playboy magazines that one of us had likely lifted from his father's collection. We kept them in the garage away from our parents' prying eyes. Mom and Pop had never been able to bring themselves to explain the birds and the bees, and in that vacuum, imagination ran wild. My friends and I had an ongoing debate: Was the meaning of 69 six seconds to f*** and nine months to get the baby, or was it six minutes? Two years later, I fancied myself expert enough that when Pop offered to buy me a book that might have corrected a few misconceptions, I turned him down.

Considering that my father was a clinical psychologist, he could be remarkably clueless as a parent. Witness (in addition to his inability to talk to his son about the facts of life) no restrictions on junk television, candy or processed food. One time, though, he surprised me. Shortly after my parents figured out I'd been smoking, when I was maybe 11, Pop appeared at my room and offered me a deal. If I agreed to quit, I wouldn't be in trouble.

I accepted the offer and never touched another cigarette.

Unfortunately, he was less successful in getting my mother to quit. Mom hadn't smoked until she was 35, when my father taught her the then-fashionable habit. Chesterfields, unfiltered. That couldn't have helped me during the pregnancy and afterwards. Nobody knew about second-hand smoke then. When I was a teenager, she'd get pissed if I opened the vent window on my side of the car to get some fresh air. When the health warnings came in the early 60s, Pop quit, but she never could. "He was hell to live with for one year," she said, and that became the justification for her never trying to stop. Eventually she switched to a lower tar and nicotine brand, but she knew how to suck on them just right to end-run the filter and get the medicine. She smoked more of them, too.

On a steamy summer day when I was 11 years old, I played tackle football with my friends on the grassy boulevard in front of our house. None of us wore helmets. That night, I turned down dinner, which never happened. Then I came down before bed and requested a bowl of shredded wheat, which also never happened. That's what Pop ate. Cap'n Crunch would have been more like it. My best guess is that I had a mild concussion.

It was one of those improbably hot nights, stuffy and still. Desperate not to hinder any breeze that might arise,

I removed the screen from my bedroom window. I slept with my head as close to the open window as possible, and at some point, I fell asleep. Next thing I knew, I found myself lying on the cement walkway two stories below. In the throes of sleep, I had fallen from the window.

Lying on the ground, I realized that I'd been dreaming. In the dream, I climbed out the window and down the drainpipe. Part way down, I figured that I could jump the rest of the way. But after I let go, I realized that I hadn't yet reached the electrical meter, mounted several feet off the ground. I shouldn't have jumped so soon. I woke from the dream when my body hit the cement.

At some point, the young couple that rented the coach house behind our home returned, probably from a bar. They spied me on the ground and decided the best thing to do was to drag me inside through the back door, where they left me.

The entire left side of my body felt bruised. It was too painful to try to make it up the stairs to my parents' bedroom, but I managed the few steps up the landing to the first floor. From there, I crawled into the living room and onto the couch, where I cried out for my parents. But the walls and doors of the house we lived in were so thick that sound didn't carry.

Perhaps half an hour later, Mom thought she heard the cat and came down to investigate, with Pop a few steps behind her. I told them, "I fell out of the window. I think I broke my wrist."

"You just had a bad dream," Mom said.

"Look," Pop said. "There's dirt on his pajama bottoms." He drove his pastel green VW bug right behind the ambulance all the way to the hospital. When it went through red lights, so did he.

———

I was still 11, when I announced to my parents that I was an atheist, and didn't want to go to church any more. They insisted that I had no choice. My best friend and next-door neighbor was another Catholic boy who by that time had zero interest in attending Mass. We used to walk in the direction of the church, until we diverted toward the Butter Bun restaurant. My friend even had a generic sermon, potentially good for any Sunday, that he'd be able to summarize if his parents quizzed him when he got home. Mine never did.

But after a while, my parents caught on, and they insisted that I attend the Sunday service with them. I sat restless in the pew as my mother prayed and sang the stolid hymns, and my father fingered his gold-embossed Italian missal. Then I had an insight: if I just got up and walked out during the service, there was no way for my parents to stop me without causing a scene.

After I did that a couple of times, my parents convened a powwow at home with me and Debbie. They announced that neither of us would be required to attend church any longer, though my sister continued to go. Interestingly, my liberation was also the beginning of Pop's release from church duty. It turned out he had as little use for it as I did, but made a show of it for the sake of my mother, who viewed it as her duty to raise us to be good Catholics. Pop's Italian Bible had been his way of entertaining himself, learning the language while the elderly Monsignor droned on.

My mother, Mary Elizabeth McCall, born a McDonald, was a force of nature. I called her "Hurricane Betty." She was a tomboy, playing sports with the boys, often her three older brothers. The name she mostly heard as a kid was "Sis," though in school she was known as Lizzie. But when it was time to go off to college, her mother thought she needed a more dignified name, so Betty it became.

Mom liked to tell the story (one of her pantheon of nearly verbatim renditions of her formative experiences) that her brothers told her that she wasn't really part of the family. She'd been found in a garbage can. She claimed to have believed this her entire childhood.

In the professionally-taken family photo circa 1919, Mom is wearing an embroidered white dress, sitting on her mother's right thigh, her little sister Helen on the left. Two older brothers stood in the back, wearing stiff suit coats and shirts with enormous starched collars. Her brother Bill was still young enough for a sailor suit. Mom stared at the camera, an adorable blond in a Prince Valiant haircut, perhaps five years old, looking pissed. Or maybe just defiant. Both words would have applied to the mother I grew up with.

She was a control freak and an alpha female who did not tolerate other strong women in her life. As fate would have it, both of my brothers married assertive women, and there were years of trouble. Mom could be a petulant three-year-old when she was mad. She'd get so upset sometimes that she and Pop, her live-in psychotherapist, would retire to the bedroom for multi-hour counseling sessions to try to calm her down.

———

My mother's father was a high school principal in New York City, the first Irish-American to achieve such a rank. The job came with a university professorship and a guaranteed annual salary of $17,000. The Irish were considered undesirable immigrants back then, but laws prevented them from being discriminated against for public sector jobs, which was how he was able to get such a good position. His salary, which he continued to receive through the Great Depression, transformed his family from middle class to wealthy. That's when he bought the farmhouse and land in Vermont, and became a gentleman farmer.

During my mother's youth, a cook prepared all the meals, and my mother wasn't allowed in the kitchen. When she married my father, it was a time when the woman was expected to assume all domestic duties, and Mom didn't know where to begin. Pop liked to tell the story that the first meal she served him was graham crackers and milk. He taught her how to cook, and judging by the results, didn't do a great job.

The food on our table wasn't just bland. The beef was roasted until there wasn't a trace of pink, the baked potatoes desiccated and the frozen peas and lima beans boiled until soggy. These were all rendered palatable with dollops of butter and salt, the only condiments my father would allow. He could say, "No onions, no garlic," in 13 languages. Pop told me, "You don't like onions and garlic," and I believed it for years.

In order to satisfy my father's demand that food have no spice whatsoever, my mother came up with a recipe for spaghetti that we ate every Friday. The sauce was made from a combination of V8 juice and Velveeta cheese. Most Catholic families ate fish on Fridays since the Church forbade the eating of meat back then, but Pop wouldn't touch fish. Once again, with enough butter and salt, the spaghetti didn't taste bad.

The only chink in his dietary control came when my brothers were home for vacations from college. They started ordering thin-crust, cheese and spicy sausage pizza from a local Italian place. Those pizzas were a revelation for Debbie and me. We started asking for them regularly instead of whatever Mom was cooking, and we succeeded often.

Otherwise, I never ate any non-Irish ethnic food until I was an adult. The only time I had seafood was when a fisherman on the lake in Vermont gave us a rainbow trout he'd caught. My mother only got me to try it by insisting — you guessed it — that it tasted just like chicken.

———————

Pop was a psychology professor and earned a respectable but not amazing salary. But Mom, who had majored in economics, was a financial whiz. Her women's Catholic college in New Jersey had allowed her to invent this major in order to keep her. When I was eight, she figured out a way we could afford to buy the former mansion of one of the lesser members of the family that owned the Schlitz brewery. The rent she charged tenants for the coach house — the former butler's quarters above the garage — more than paid for the mortgage and taxes, which meant that we lived there for free.

We went from a modest starter house near the University of Wisconsin-Milwaukee, with no room to spare, to a cavernous mansion on Newberry Boulevard. It had an intercom system with little flags that would pop up to indicate to the servants (which we did not have) which room had rung. There were floor-to-ceiling mirrors in the bathrooms, laundry chutes, and cut-glass chandeliers. Pop raved about Mom's cleverness with money, although, as usual, his praise would have been delivered outside her earshot.

Whatever his overall opinion was, Pop always led with the negative. He would praise you, you might later learn, but never to your face. To Debbie and me he would say,

"Your mother is such a strong swimmer," but as she did the crawl in front of our dock at the lake house, he'd yell, "Get your left hand out of the water!" Mom kept swimming without any perceptible change in how high she lifted that hand.

––––––––––

Mom loved it when people called her "a character." She was the only female carpenter anyone had ever heard of, or so went the running joke among my father's fellow professors at Marquette University. I remember getting my mother a hammer one Christmas. She couldn't have been more pleased.

When I was 12, Mom, Debbie and I, along with a 17-year-old foster kid named Al, built a two-room extension on the Vermont lake house. I hammered the floorboards and shingled parts of the roof. My sister painted the walls. My mother did the electrical wiring. That house and addition are still standing.

Mom-the-carpenter fit right into the male culture in the house. All three of the children my mother gave birth to were boys. Of all the foster kids we had over the years, all but one were boys. Although my father had a soft side, he was an alpha male at work, and he had grown up as a scrappy handball player on the streets of the Bronx. Pop used to say that his father, a fire captain in Greenwich Village, "could knock a man out with a single punch" — and if any of his men hit their wives, he took them out back for a beating. Even our pets were almost exclusively male, and we had dozens of them over the years. Just as with the foster kids, it was Mom who chose all the animals. The only female pet I remember was one of three kittens we'd found abandoned in a cardboard box. I named them after my basketball hero, then the center on the Milwaukee Bucks: Kareem, Abdul, and Jabbar. The female was Abdul.

Pop told me several times that his vocabulary was the largest of anyone he had ever met. He was one of the last of a generation who learned Latin and Greek in school, so he knew any word derived from them. He wasn't a show-off about it, just precise, and he loathed it when others used words in pompous ways that he judged to be incorrect. As we watched Monday Night Football, he would ridicule Howard Cosell who thought it was erudite to call a fistfight on the field an altercation.

Starting when I was 10, Pop encouraged me to watch football games with him. During his college years he had been two years ahead of Vince Lombardi at Fordham, who went on to coach the Green Bay Packers — our local team. Watching football was my best opportunity to bond with Pop, who was otherwise too busy with his work and other interests. Many evenings I convinced him to play catch with me with a mini-football in the upstairs hall next to the pool table. If I jumped high and snagged a pass, he sometimes clapped and congratulated me, and I took great joy in that.

I found watching the Packers addictive because the team was so good. I even kept a scrapbook for a while. The first year I watched The Pack, as we called them, they won the NFL championship. The second year they won the first Super Bowl. The third year they did it again. Then they sucked for a long, long time.

Pop himself was on TV. He had a regular segment on psychology called The Mind's Eye on the local daytime hit, *Dialing for Dollars*. The show was co-hosted by the station's weatherman and his wife. Pop was also interviewed regularly on the news for a psychological perspective on current events, particularly when someone had committed a heinous crime.

In our family you were never in trouble until you had a chance to talk your way out of it. Everything was debated. The dinner table was an intellectual Roman Coliseum with Pop as Caesar, rendering thumbs up or down. I still remember how validated I felt when he sided with me when I was maybe six, telling Tony (with whom I was disagreeing) that I had made a good point. In our family there wasn't much physical or verbal affection, so this kind of attention — unfortunately often at someone else's expense — was the best you could get.

Ultra-competitive in everything he did, even with his own children, Pop regularly tried to "win the point" while we were warming up in tennis. He did the same to my mother, who wasn't a strong player. And he showed no mercy to me and Debbie when we played the word-spelling game Ghost during the winter-break drives to Florida and the two-day trips between Vermont and Milwaukee that book-ended the summer. Each player adds a letter, trying not to complete a word. You would think you finally had him, but he would triumphantly announce some unexpected letter. Stumped, we'd challenge him, and he'd pronounce some word we'd never heard of, providing definitions and sometimes etymology.

———

Pop came by his competitive nature honestly, a family legacy from his father and their shared pitta nature. They used to arm wrestle regularly, and my grandfather always won. One day when Pop was a young man, they engaged in a protracted struggle and finally Pop pinned his father's arm. The next day his father, then 64, suffered a heart attack.

On his deathbed a week later, he told his wife, my grandmother, that he thought it had been the arm-wrestling that had precipitated the attack. His mother mentioned it to Pop in the weeks after his father died, which, as Ray puts it, "Must have felt like a dagger from the grave." I learned this story from Ray, who heard it from Mom. Pop never spoke of it to us.

Strangely, Pop almost never spoke of his mother either, other than to say she died of a rare duodenal cancer. I know nothing more about her, and never thought to ask until it was too late. It wasn't until a few years ago that a cousin told me her first name — Nell. She also told me that Nell was the first woman in Texas to be photographed riding a bicycle, the kind with a giant front wheel, and a tiny back wheel. That piece of information raised more questions than it answered, but I was thrilled to learn it.

I always feared Pop's anger. That's probably how I started to develop the interpersonal radar that has proved useful in my life. If he came home in a foul mood, I'd get one whiff of it and head straight for my room and start straightening it up. If I got enough time before he arrived at my door looking for a fight, he'd step inside, scan the room and, seeing nothing to bitch about, harrumph and storm off to find another target.

If Pop found the basement light on when he rose at 5:00 a.m., he'd march first to my room, snap on the overhead light, and ask me if I was responsible. If I was, he made me get up, go down to the basement and turn it off. If I pleaded ignorance, Debbie's light would go on next.

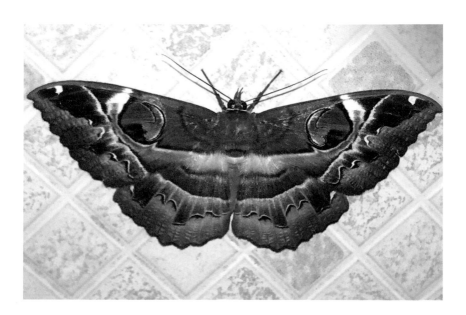

When I was a kid, the release of every new Beatles album was an event. I had just turned 12, and Ray had brought home their latest LP, Sgt. Pepper's Lonely Hearts Club Band. The family gathered in the living room around Pop's stereo, housed in the built-in cabinet that Mom had fashioned. This ceremonial unveiling was part of Ray's ongoing effort to convince Pop that the Beatles were actually good.

Pop, who favored Mozart, had to admit that "Yesterday," which the band had released two years earlier, wasn't bad, but he remained skeptical after the first few songs on Sgt. Pepper's. As Ringo sang "With A Little Help from My Friends," Pop asked, "Is he intentionally singing out of tune?"

By then, Ray had flunked out of college twice, and was singing and playing lead guitar and keyboards for a Milwaukee rock band called The Shags. They'd turned a basement bar, once a bowling alley, into the city's hottest night spot. They were the first long-haired, all-original music group in the city, and we were all thrilled when they were given a recording contract by Capitol Records, the same label as the Beatles. Ray's song, "Stop and Listen" became the band's first and only single for the label. He sang lead, in his best Mick Jagger growl, and played fuzz-tone guitar. That song was played on my favorite radio station many times a day.

After the 45 was released, Ray and the band were invited to perform "Stop and Listen" "live" on a local TV show, which I watched at home. They weren't supposed to actually play the song, just lip-synch it, while mock-playing their instruments. They all thought this was stupid, so they hatched a plan. Ray mouthed the words with great emotion, but as a put-on, the band had brought instruments not featured on the recording, and as the record spun, they pretended to play them. The drummer left his kit unused and blew into a flute. The rhythm guitarist bowed a violin. Ray sneaked an autoharp (a member of the zither family) onto the soundstage, hidden under his leather cape. He took it out mid-song, just in time for his dramatic air-guitar solo. The performance left me in stitches. All my friends at school knew about The Shags. Watching Ray do all of this was the coolest thing ever.

My parents had been involved in the civil rights movement. When it was time to think about high school, though, they told me I could go to any school I wanted except for the nearest public school, which was predominantly African-American. Although it was walking distance from the house and seemed like an obvious choice, it had a bad reputation. This meant Catholic school was my only option.

I'd enjoyed the third grade in Catholic school, when I'd had a warm-hearted, young woman as a teacher, who, as I recall, had recently been married. In my school photo from that year, I'm glowing. Otherwise, I hated my time in Catholic elementary school. First grade was the worst, but a couple of other nuns, particularly one I had in sixth grade, were awful. She was so bad that my mother let me transfer to a public school for the remainder of grade school. It was so much better. When it was time for high school, I did not want to go to another parochial school. The local Catholic boys' prep school was my parents' first choice, though, and I agreed to take the entrance exam, an all-day affair held at the school.

As I stood in the cafeteria line on the day of the exam, a boy asked me if I would go to the prom with him. I had started growing my hair out several months earlier. By then, it was still shorter than the Fab Four's on the *Beatles '65* album cover — already more than five years old — but it was longer than any boy's hair at the school. In that politically polarized time, with anti-Vietnam War hippies on one side and Nixon's "silent majority" on the other, long hair was a cultural and political statement. I told the boy that I was sorry to decline his generous offer, but I wasn't gay.

While I was still in the lunch line, a man with a whistle around his neck approached me. He demanded to know if I was a boy or a girl. This was familiar territory to me — by then, I'd heard that question dozens of times. I knew there was never any genuine doubt.

I was four foot ten and weighed 85 pounds — and this gym teacher, or whatever he was, towered over me — but I wasn't going to take any sh*t from him. "How many girls take this test?" I said.

"Don't beat around the bush."

"I'm a boy."

"The next time you come back here, you look like one," he said, and handed me the school handbook with a paper clip on the dress code page.

It was a deal. I never returned.

I ended up at attending a Catholic high school in a suburb dubbed "White Folks Bay." My hair proved to be a problem there, too. A few of my classmates threatened to hold me down and cut it off. My biology teacher interrupted a lecture to ask, "Do you even own a comb?" One nun, a sweet but ineffectual soul, told me she thought it was good I was there, so that people could see that someone could have long hair and still be clean. I concluded that it would be good if I weren't there at all, for any reason.

After listening to my complaints for one semester, my parents reluctantly allowed me to transfer to the public high school. It was a tough environment, but I learned a lot about real life there. Girls brought their babies to class. There were robberies in the hall, which, at my size, I endured regularly. "Hey man, give me a quarter," was the common refrain. Drug deals and blowjobs went down in the bathrooms. The buzz among the students was that one of the vice principals was "a narc," an undercover narcotics agent. I remember hearing that at any one time, one third of the students were absent. Few of my classmates went on to college. At least no one hassled me about my hair.

This was the age when I decided that I wanted to be called Timothy and not Tim — though my family is still working on that one. I liked the sound of Timothy better. But I bet I was also influenced by my black classmates. I remember a kid in my homeroom who corrected the teacher taking attendance: His name was Charles — not Chuck.

I hung out with proto-hoodlums until their misdemeanors gave way to breaking and entering and joyriding in stolen cars. One day I was walking home from school when a few friends pulled alongside me in a car. I got in the back seat between two of them. As we rode along, the driver, someone I'd never seen before, repeatedly yanked the stick shift on steering column into reverse, rocking the car to a stop. "Tranny drops," he called them. I felt sorry for the poor sucker who owned the car.

I knew it was time to move on. I started hanging around with a different group of kids, instead. We met every morning before school in an attic bedroom to listen to "Black Magic Woman," and "Sympathy for the Devil." As the bong passed from hand to hand around the room, we coughed, one by one, in circular sequence.

―――――――

"You look like Mary Travers," Pop said. By that time, around age 17, my straight blonde hair hung down to the middle of my back. I'd grown up singing three-part harmonies of Peter, Paul and Mary songs with Tony and Ray, so he knew I'd get the allusion.

Over the years, Pop and I fought many battles over my hair, and at first he "pulled rank," as he put it. But after a while he gave up on that tack and moved on to the "gentle" art of persuasion (as always, tinged with insult).

"Ray has long hair," I argued. "Why can't I?"

"He needs it for his work," Pop said. That was the lamest excuse I'd ever heard.

―――――――

I think Pop wanted Tony to stick it to (what he perceived to be) the snobs at the country club in Vermont by winning the annual men's tennis tournament. Ever the scrappy Irish kid, he likely felt judged by the well-to-do WASPs that populated the club, many of whom, Pop pointed out, had "last names for first names." Located in a more upscale town nearby, the club was the only place in the area where we could play tennis. Tony was on his college tennis team, but he wasn't quite good enough to bring home the hardware Pop coveted.

Once I came along, my father saw to it that I was groomed from an earlier age. He taught Debbie and me when we were little, sometimes reducing us to tears on the club's red clay courts. One time during a lesson, he got so angry with me for some offense (which I can no longer recall) that he chased me around the club, wielding his steel T2000 tennis racket like a cudgel, but I evaded him. Starting when I was around 12, he sprang for weekly private tennis lessons in the indoor club he played at in Milwaukee.

And then one year in my late twenties, I did it — I won the championship at the country club, after my opponent's drop shot on match point hit the top of the net and fell back on his side. In the Polaroid someone snapped afterwards, my opponent, Tom, a consummate gentleman who had beaten me every time we'd played on his way to winning prior years' tournaments, smiles warmly. I'm standing next to him, wearing a headband that I tore from an old white towel, tied around my scruffy blond hair. I hold a pewter bowl in my hand, beaming. It had been a singular focus of mine to win that tournament for as long as I could remember. It would be years before I realized that it was a goal that Pop had implanted in my consciousness.

When Mom and I walked in the door of the lake house after we got home from the club, the phone was ringing. It was Pop, calling from California. The timing was just a

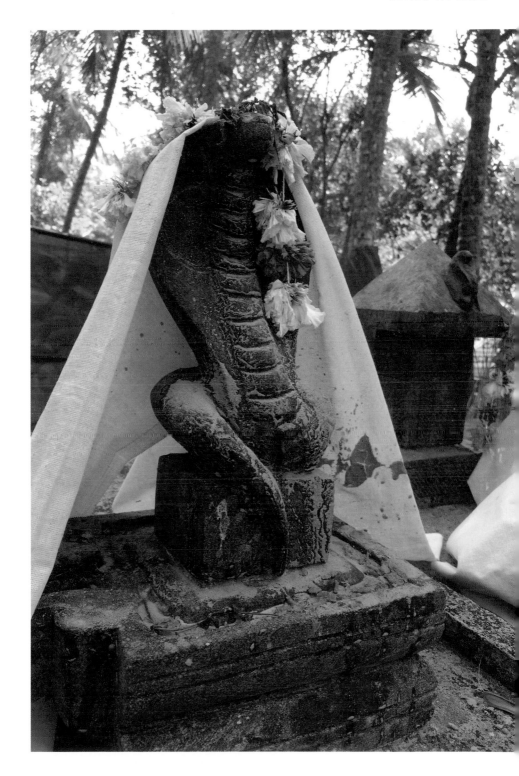

coincidence, he claimed — he was on a break at the psychology convention he was attending. If he was thrilled about my victory, he didn't let it on to me.

I was a good tennis player, but not as good as I might have been. I had all the shots. The form on my strokes was excellent. But my mind often got in the way. I was a master at wrestling defeat from the jaws of victory. I'd be way up in a match but could not hold onto the lead. The closer I got to winning, the more anxious I got. Presumably, on some level I didn't believe I deserved to win, though I would not have been able to articulate that.

I suffered from what tennis players call an "iron elbow." When the game was close or I was in the lead, I'd get tight and be unable to make the shots that were usually easy for me. Then I'd get frustrated and put more pressure on myself, which only made matters worse. I'd berate myself, swear and throw rackets. All of this brought me great shame. It was only after I'd practiced the inner game of tennis for several years that I was able to overcome my performance anxiety and learned to play better than usual on big points. That's what allowed me to finally win the club championship.

While Tony's strokes were unorthodox, he knew how to win. He and I played a few hard-fought matches, and my recollection is that he won more than I did. But win or lose, those outings (which started when I was a teenager) were excruciating for me. I hated the pressure and strangeness of battling my big brother. I suspect he must have felt something similar because, without ever discussing it, we stopped playing sets, and whenever we went out on the court, we simply hit the ball without keeping score. That was actually fun.

Pop was a dapper dresser, at least in his own mind. He almost always wore a suit jacket with a pocket square, even at the grocery store and the dry cleaners, where he insisted on being called Dr. McCall. He was a metrosexual, long before the term existed. He wore cologne and garter belts on his calves to hold up his socks, common among men of that era. But some of his behavior was unusual. He used cuticle pushers and special pencils to whiten his nails. He once shaved his armpits because he said he thought it was more hygienic. He refused to use public urinals because of the smell, and once told me that he would never go to India, which he considered to be "a cesspool."

We kids thought his polka dot shirts and ascots were absurd. I was mortified by his tennis outfits, with matching shirt, socks, and shorts, either yellow or powder blue. He ridiculed hippie fashion, but after a couple of women told him how good he looked when he dressed as a "freak" for a Halloween party, the Revolution was on. By Monday morning he had a whole new wardrobe with big-collared shirts and flared trousers — though he never went all the way to bell bottoms, the only pants I ever wore. I think the polka dots must have been an attempt to be "far out," though it never occurred to me at the time.

My father was much harder on my brothers than he was on me. Ray and Pop, aka Raymond Joseph McCall Jr. and Sr., never got along. Pop was overseas during World War II when Ray Jr. was born. When Ray was three, a strange man moved in and started bossing them around. They never fully recovered from that rocky start.

Pop had been an academic superstar. He'd won the award as the top senior at Fordham, beating out former CIA director Bill Casey. Pop had two PhDs, one in

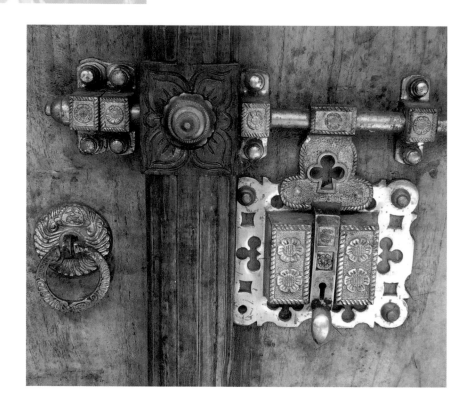

philosophy and the other in psychology, and became a professor at St. John's in New York in his mid-twenties. For years, he was the Chairman of the department of psychology at Marquette, and wrote books and articles in his field. Ray Jr., after his slow start, finally ended up resuscitating his flagging academic career by landing a position in an architecture PhD program, and eventually he became a professor of environmental design.

"I am the failed prototype for Ray Jr.," he says. "Tony is the successful implementation."

"You had enormously more choice and freedom than we had," Ray tells me. Pop's initial infatuation with his last hostage to fortune, he says, "slowly segued into making half-hearted attempts to rein you in." Ray was a rebel like me, but Tony, the middle child, took another tack. "Tony followed every rule they made," Ray says, in what he calls "Catholic North Korea."

Tony went to medical school, because that was Pop's agenda for him. (Pop had the same plan for me, and although I resisted for a couple of years, I eventually relented. I couldn't tell if my lingering doubts were coming from my inner wisdom, or simply in response to his not-so-subtle attempts to push me.) After his medical residency, Tony served as chief resident and then did an endocrinology fellowship at the same Boston medical center. After that, Tony pursued a PhD in neuron and endocrine studies. He got straight A's in grad school, and suffered through years of working with a thesis adviser who Ray describes as a "power-tripping monster." At his graduation ceremony, Tony told Ray, "This is the last thing I ever have to do for Pop." The successful prototype was now positioned to ascend the ladder of academic medicine.

Later on that evening, when they were celebrating Tony's graduation, Pop mentioned to Tony and Ray that I'd just made Phi Beta Kappa at Wisconsin. By that time, Ray was finishing up his own PhD. I'd found the invitation to join the honor society weeks after it had been sent, buried in a pile of junk mail. It was on the dining room table of my house in Madison, right next to a bong and a bag of pot that my roommates permanently left there. "That Tim," Pop said, "he's the real scholar in the family."

At Mom and Pop's 50th wedding anniversary celebration at the Vermont farmhouse, I performed a song I wrote. The chorus went:

Who left the light on in the basement?
Who left the dog out in the yard?
Who left the back door wide open?
We're not paying to heat Newberry Boulevard!

That last line didn't quite scan but I couldn't change it, because the exact wording of each of the lines had been etched, like water carving the Grand Canyon, into the neural circuitry of every member of the family.

As usual, Mom was parked in her armchair next to the phone in the farmhouse dining room the night of that celebration. The rest of the family, including Pop, sat around the weathered wood table, covered with an intricate cloth that she had crocheted. A few more relatives sprawled on the antique horsehair couch.

At the dinner, held in a restaurant a few towns over, everyone's eyes were riveted on Pop. We kids had become suspicious that he might be developing Alzheimer's and that Mom had been covering it up. With them down in Florida, where they'd moved after Pop retired, it was hard to know.

Two years earlier, at a family gathering in Tony and Madelyn's backyard, I began to think that Pop might have early dementia. He'd made a comment to me, which I no longer recall. All I remember is that it made perfect sense, but it was simply something that the Raymond J. McCall I knew would never have said. I shared my suspicions with Tony, but the mere suggestion made him angry. He could not even consider that my claim might have some truth.

At the 50th anniversary dinner, and in numerous conversations that day, Pop had seemed fine. He told stories about Mom and himself in animated detail. As the night wound down, after what had been a long eventful day, we were all sitting around in the dim light from an overhead fixture in the farm house dining room. Pop leaned across the table and said to Tony, "So, what do *you* do for a living?"

I felt like I'd been punched in the stomach. It had to have been a lot worse for Tony.

The next day, Tony drove Pop down from Vermont to Boston, where he and Madelyn were still living, to be evaluated. The doctors did all the routine tests and no treatable causes for his mental decline were found. This left Alzheimer's disease as the presumptive diagnosis, and foretold an inevitable decline in his functioning.

Pop had been a turbo-charged intellectual machine, and the faculty taken from him was his brain. Back in Vermont in the weeks after his diagnosis, he told me that he only had "a mild case of Alzheimer's." The denial in that comment mirrored the punch line of a joke I'd heard him tell dozens of times, in which a young woman confronted by her parents finally admits that she is "slightly pregnant."

As my father descended into the oblivion of dementia over the next three years, he developed a fever of unknown cause and was hospitalized at a private hospital near my parents' home in Florida. Although the fever abated with antibiotics, the hospital stay had not gone well. Mom told me that a nurse, frustrated with feeding him, had taken it on herself to cut off his beard without permission. According to his roommate, aides had to hold Pop down as she shaved it off.

After finishing a couple of shifts I'd committed to at the medical clinic where I worked, I flew from Boston into West Palm Beach. Mom told me that Pop no longer recognized her and hadn't spoken in over three months. I visited him that day. The hospital was sleek, with modern art and well-tended plants in the lobby.

After spending awhile in Pop's room, I wandered over to the nurses' station. Without asking for permission, I walked up to the rack of patients' charts and removed my father's. I sat down at the nurses' station to read. It soon became clear that the hospital was doing nothing for him. Various consultants had left one-line notes from time to time. He was supposedly getting daily speech therapy, which could not possibly have helped him.

The next day, I arranged for his discharge. Mom and I rented a hospital bed and set it up in the living room. My foster brother Pat, a registered nurse and career Army officer, flew in from the other side of the country to help minister to Pop at home.

Pop was groggy when I entered his hospital room. His cheeks were sunken, covered in stubble. Wearing only a hospital gown, he was lying back with the head of the bed raised. I greeted him but he didn't respond.

I had brought a portable music player and headphones, with a tape of his favorite piece of music, a Mozart violin concerto. I placed the headset over his ears and pressed play. After a few seconds, he lifted his head and cocked it to one side like he'd just had a good idea. "It's beautiful," he whispered.

Mom was holding Pop's hand three weeks later when he let out his last breath.

When Mom would come to Vermont for the summer in the years after Pop's death, she stayed at the farmhouse. By this time, I was the only member of the family who still used the lake house. I was lucky if I could get her down to the water even once in the season for a swim.

As with every home my mother had, the lake house contained two houses' worth of furniture. Some of her possessions were beautiful: unrecognized antiques she gotten for a few dollars at Goodwill or St. Vincent De-Paul, or furniture from the occasional estate sale. The treasures, though, were always mixed in with junk. She rarely threw anything out. A plastic day-glow-orange flower arrangement, in which several petals and a couple of stems had broken off, sat on a marble-top bureau next to a gorgeous 19th century clock.

In Debbie's old room in the lake house were a couple of ancient twin beds made of steel. Dilapidated mattresses that stank of mildew rested on built-in metal springs. One summer, while Mom was still down in Florida, I decided those mattresses had to go.

Steve, the guy in town who'd been the caretaker of the properties, and whom my mother was fond of, helped me load them into the back of his pickup. This wasn't easy because they had the consistency of overcooked lasagna noodles. We drove down the lumber road on the farm property to a clearing where we burned them. Three years later, Mom still hadn't forgiven me.

Mom died when she was 91. Between my birth and three weeks before her death, she spent a total of one day in the hospital. I called her program the "Betty Mc-Call two-pack-a-day longevity plan." Sadly, she did what most members of her family had before her: she died bitter. She'd had every advantage in life. But in her final years, she was fuming at the world, a cigarette with a long-hanging column of ash poised between her tobacco-stained fingers.

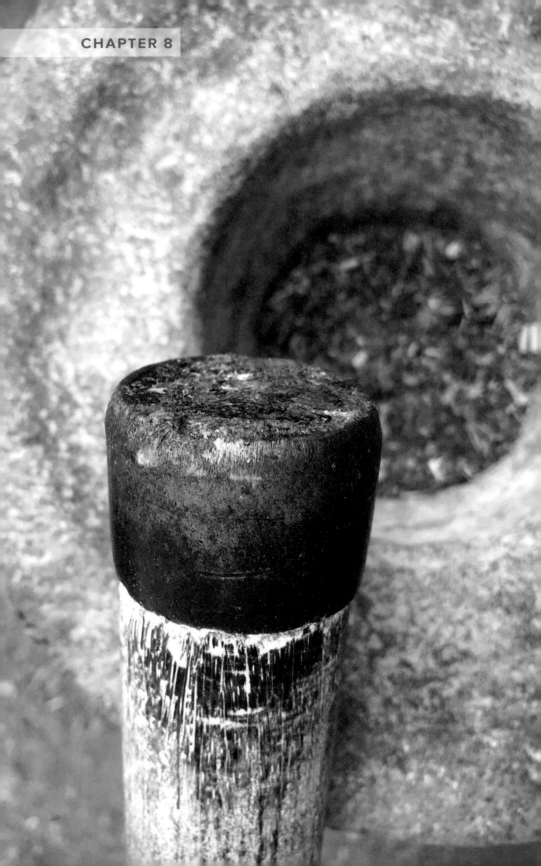

NAVEL GAZING

Reading through my baby book at home in Burlington, I came across a photo of myself, taken when I was eight days old. I never would have recognized myself if it hadn't been mounted in that album. The newborn me looks terrified. What's most striking is the tension in my tiny hands. They are held up, tendons stretched taut, like the claws of a cat prepared to strike.

For years, I've been aware that I hold a lot of tension in my hands. Sometimes when I feel relaxed, I notice my fingers are curled into fists — for no reason I can discern. By directing my attention there, I get them to let go, but later I often discover that I'm clenching them again.

I've suspected for a long time that this habit started in the incubator — I must have felt petrified and isolated. It seems likely that I was stuck with a lot of needles in my first month outside the womb. Furthermore, the effect of maternal smoking on the newborn was still unrecognized at that time. Research has found that nicotine-exposed infants showed hyper-aroused nervous systems and other signs of drug withdrawal similar to crack babies. That freaked-out infant was probably being flooded with stress hormones, which would have resulted in a major increase in the vata dosha, associated in Ayurveda with fear. I'd long since intuited that both my long-standing vata derangement and my twitchy nervous system started early. This photograph is the first evidence I've seen that supports this idea.

At the time of my birth, it was believed that physical contact with babies could be harmful to their development. Hospitals cautioned against touching infants any more than necessary. In an incubator, babies would have been handled even less, perhaps only when held to be fed a bottle or to have their diapers changed.

This was before Dr. Harry Harlow's research at the University of Wisconsin's Primate Laboratory. He studied baby rhesus monkeys deprived of motherly love and affection. In one infamous study, monkeys that were separated from their mothers at birth, and raised alone in cages, were given a choice between two surrogate mothers. One was made of wire but had a milk bottle attached. The other was covered in soft terry cloth, which was heated by a light from behind, but had no bottle.

Behaviorists believed that it was the food the mother provides that reinforces the infant's bond with her. They would have predicted that the baby monkeys would favor the wire surrogate. That is the opposite of what happened. The monkeys showed a strong preference for the soft mothers, hugging them, clinging to them, sleeping at their feet. They spent just enough time on the wire surrogates to drink the milk then scampered back to their terry cloth moms.

Ironically, it was Harlow's own experiments that

demonstrated just how inhumane depriving infant primates of maternal love and contact could be: they wound up with severe deficits in cognitive function and social behavior. While initially celebrated, his research was later castigated, and it is believed to have been instrumental in the development of the animal rights movement.

As fate would have it, I wound up as a psychology major at the University of Wisconsin. One of my professors worked at the primate lab founded by Harlow, though I was not involved with it. A friend, though, had a part-time job there. He called it "Monkey State Penitentiary."

When I was a happy-go-lucky toddler, Pop used to refer to me as "jug ears" and seemed to delight in it. I laughed, too, not that I understood that much better than when he called me his "last hostage to fortune." I knew he thought my ears were large but I never worried about it. Looking back at photos, I can see that they stuck out to the sides.

Twenty years later, I was sitting in a barber's chair in Madison, Wisconsin, instructing the woman to leave the hair long over my ears. I admitted to her that I usually kept them covered because they were so large. She combed the hair back on either side and said, "No they're not."

On a sunny day soon thereafter, I walked past several brown and white jugs on display in front of an antique shop. I looked at the jugs' handles and for the first time in my life I understood the nickname. I remember thinking, *F*** you, Pop!* Looking back, I don't think his intention was to be mean, but there was often a cutting edge to his humor.

Pop coined a psychological term, "defensive devaluation," which is the act of putting someone else down to build yourself up. In the textbook he wrote, *The Varieties of Abnormality*, he described it as a self-protective maneuver in which one focuses "on the weaknesses and aberrations of others as a means of diverting attention from one's own deficiencies and lapses." The defensive devaluator, he wrote, "does not criticize in the hope of effecting reform but as a defense against his own sense of inadequacy and perhaps guilt." I don't think he realized how much this description applied to him. As he wrote, "He sees the mote in his neighbor's eye but misses the splinter in his own, and with a vengeance."

I didn't see it as a kid, but I've come to realize that Pop could be a supercilious prick. He was a master of a tactic I call "winning through humiliation." In early adulthood, I realized I had inadvertently modeled some of Pop's hypercritical behavior, employing what I dubbed "McCall verbal assassin mode" — humor at someone else's expense. I soon figured out it was a profoundly anti-social skill, and gave it up. Early in their careers, Tony and Ray had similar epiphanies.

Pop's sharp tongue cost him in his professional life. It didn't help that he was a fierce critic of both the leading school in academic psychology at the time, behaviorism, and the dominant influence in psychiatry, Freudian theory. He'd ridicule someone's ideas at a conference or a committee meeting at school, winning the day — and making an enemy for life. He was devastated when several of his fellow professors banded together and ousted him from his position as Chairman of the Psychology Department at Marquette. Like his other defeats, he never talked about it — and never forgot.

Mom could be charming and entertaining. She'd taught herself Ragtime piano and played at parties. People outside the family, though, couldn't see the signs that all was not well. Though she never spoke of it, Ray and I figured out that she had significant phobias: of heights, of flying, of caterpillars. Mom had a temper, and if you got on her bad side — as I watched my brothers and sister do at different times after they'd moved out the house — you might be paying for it for years. There were long spells of little to no communication between her and each of my siblings during their adult years.

I escaped the consequences of her long-term grudges, but as a teenager we butted heads — especially when she figured out, when I was maybe 16, that my friends and I smoked pot. She started reading reefer-madness articles in *Reader's Digest*. Overnight, she went from being clueless to haranguing me when I returned home: "Why are your eyes so red and glassy?" In my way, I was as defiant as she was. That was the beginning of a difficult year.

As an adult, I forged as close a relationship with her as she was capable of — but I was frustrated with how shallow that seemed to be. Any attempt I made at emotional intimacy was deflected. She didn't seem interested in my life.

One year, during every one of our regular phone calls, I made a point to tell her about my girlfriend, who was pursuing a career as a jazz vocalist. I knew Mom would never ask, and I wanted her to know. They had met and got along fine, but she just wasn't on Mom's radar. My mother would listen politely to anything I said about my girlfriend, but never asked any questions.

For years, I heard Mom complain that her own mother had been enamored of her first grandchild — and none of the others. Yet, when the time came, she recapitulated this pattern precisely. She was ecstatic after the first of Ray's three children was born. She wasn't much interested when the others, including Tony and Madelyn's kids, came along. I've never seen a woman less invested in her grandchildren than my mother. She'd send cards on their birthdays and Christmas, but that was about it.

"We were always such a close family," Mom said multiple times, and I think she believed it. I never knew how to respond.

———————

While I was a medical resident, Mom, Pop, and I were relaxing around the table after a satisfying meal at Tony

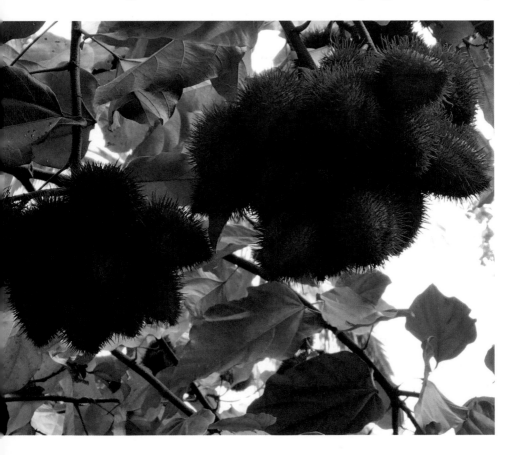

and Madelyn's suburban Boston house. Upstairs, their newborn Christopher slept. Chris started to whimper, then sob. Mom was saying how important she felt it was to let babies cry themselves back to sleep — she couldn't stand it when parents felt obligated to respond.

Madelyn listened politely but as the bawling escalated, her face reddened and she began to squirm in her seat. Finally, she let out a yelp and ran up the stairs. A short while later, Christopher settled down and Madelyn rejoined the group. In perfect Irish Catholic style, no one mentioned what had just happened.

Ten years later, on a plane ride to Oregon to take a vacation with Tony and Madelyn and their young sons, I read a book called *The Artist's Way*. This was 1995, the year I started to practice asana. The author, Julia Cameron, described a practice she called "morning pages," which she promised would change your life. I thought, *Yeah, right.*

To do morning pages, you write whatever comes into your mind in a stream of consciousness fashion, without pausing. The pen is never supposed to stop moving. If you're stuck, you can scribble, "It's cold out today," or "This ink is blue." It's important to write about whatever comes into your mind, and not censor yourself. Cameron recommends three pages longhand every day, first thing every morning after waking up.

In healthy sleepers, writing immediately after awakening would mean it would come directly after early-morning rapid eye movement (REM) sleep. That's when dreaming is typically most vivid. Studies have found that this is a fertile time for intuitive leaps and creative thinking. Perhaps for similar reasons, starting around three quarters of an hour before dawn is the period that yogis believe is the best to meditate.

Tony, Madelyn, Chris, Jon and I stayed in a rented house on a ranch in the high desert near Bend. As soon as I woke up the first morning, I got out a notebook and began to write. The results shocked me. I had scribbled three pages about my childhood. Some of this might have been triggered by a book I had read the week before, *The Drama of the Gifted Child*, by the psychologist Alice Miller. In it, she described parents who, rather than attending to their children's psychological needs, used their offspring to meet their own. So much of what she described rang true to my experience. That would be the first of many books on narcissism I would read.

The pen moved rapidly across the page, and I found myself wondering why my parents had taken in so many additional foster kids. It made no sense. Mom and Pop were too distracted by their own busy lives to pay much attention to Debbie and me. Some of those kids were dangerous. Why did my Mom keep saying yes? My theory was that it was an example of what I called the "Catholic martyr" role that she seemed to enjoy playing. Whether my speculation was right or wrong, it had never occurred to me before to even ask such questions. Doing so became an important step on my path to greater self-understanding.

Later that morning, I asked Tony about his memories of my childhood. Nine-and-a-half years my senior, he was able to fill in a few details I'd forgotten or was too young to have remembered, but he was as clueless as I was about why Mom and Pop took in so many disturbed kids. Listening to our conversation, Madelyn offered an outsider's perspective on the family. She spoke about her run-ins with Mom — she felt that she hadn't been treated fairly. And whatever Pop's flaws were, she also saw his sweet side. Madelyn had felt welcomed into the family by him, but not so much by her. Her perspective ran counter to the mostly unspoken family story that Pop was the weirdo and Mom, relatively speaking, the normal one.

I wrote morning pages every day that week, and each time I had at least one epiphany. After the conversation with Madelyn, I thought about the family mythology about my parents, and started to see that the reality was more complicated. I considered how angry and controlling Mom could be, how incapable she seemed of any true intimacy.

It occurred to me that this freeform writing was allowing me to tap into my subconscious in a way that had previously been inaccessible to me. On two occasions in the prior decade, I had done weekly psychotherapy for a year, once with a psychologist and once with a social worker. I learned more from a week of morning pages than in two years of therapy.

I wrote morning pages religiously for a long time, and still do it intermittently. Now if I sense something is brewing beneath the surface, I get out my notebook and write to figure out what it is — often with success. Other times, I'll have no idea there's something on my mind, only to discover I've just written two-and-a-half pages on it.

———————————

One of the main purposes of meditation — which doesn't get as much press as such physiological benefits as lowering blood pressure and improving immune function — is that it puts you in touch with your subconscious mind. Yoga studied this realm thousands of years before Freud supposedly invented the idea. When you get quiet in meditation, which can take years of practice, unexpected thoughts start to bubble to the surface.

Practicing yoga built my ability to look within. Yoga enhances proprioception, being able to feel where the body parts are in space even with your eyes closed, and interoception, awareness of sensations from the inner body. But over time yoga also allows practitioners to plumb the depths of their psychological states. The poses and breathing techniques help, but meditation is considered to be the most important tool in building awareness — including an awareness of the subconscious mind.

About ten years ago, a couple years after Mom had died, I was surprised to find myself further re-evaluating our relationship. I had been frustrated that I hadn't been able to form a deeper bond with her, but I didn't think it had affected me that much.

Seeing my mother's limitations more clearly, I began to realize how profoundly I must have been wounded. At first, I had to approach it intellectually. I couldn't access any related emotions. If anyone had asked me during most of my life, I would have said I'd had a happy childhood. As I began this excavation project, I had to imagine what it must have been like to be a baby with a cold, emotionally-withholding mother. Here was a woman, I suspected, who was unable to tell what her crying infant needed — and perhaps not even interested in finding out — since, as I had heard her tell Madelyn, she believed in letting babies cry themselves to sleep.

Over the next few years, I came into a deeper awareness of myself through meditation, morning pages, and ongoing psychological exploration inspired by books I had read — including both eastern and western takes on psychology. I saw that I had used every kind of fun and stimulation — sports, travel, music, cannabis, parties, dancing, romance, sex (and, yes, oral sex, too) to distract me from the pain buried deep inside. I was always focused

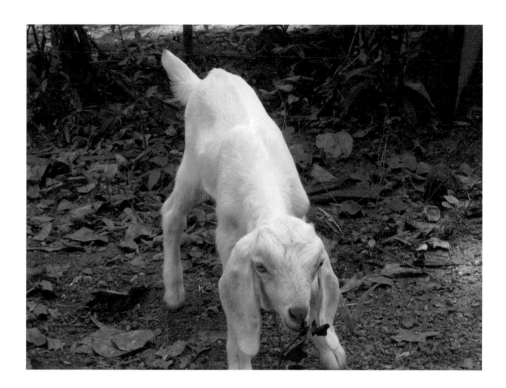

on planning the next adventure, allowing no time and no energy to look back and reflect.

Slowly, I started to access feelings that I had walled off. As I sat cross-legged during my morning meditation, which I was doing for an hour every day, I felt at different times sadness, fear, anger and shame related to my child-hood experiences. It took me a few years to work through most of it.

Eventually, I got to a place where I could forgive my mother for her limitations. I saw that she, too, was a victim of her karma. I can't know what happened in her family, but there seemed to have been a lot of suffering. Two of her three brothers had become alcoholics. Her only sister died a broken woman. Mom wasn't a bad per-son. She didn't abuse me. She provided for me materially in every way she could. She just didn't know how to give me the love I craved. Likely, she was too distracted by her endless carpentry, crochet, and reupholstery projects — and the inner turmoil, which I've come to believe that those projects were meant to keep at bay — to pay close attention to my needs.

That said, she was a vigilant, caring parent when she became aware that there was a crisis. When I suffered a head injury in a hit-and-run at age five, two blocks from where we lived, she hadn't even been aware that I'd left the house. I don't remember the accident itself, though I do have an image etched in memory of the chrome grill of a black car. I don't know if I lost consciousness, although I heard that the young woman who rescued me from the street got blood all over her dress. I also recall the nurses at the hospital not letting me fall asleep, as they were presumably worried I might drop into a coma. When my friend rang the doorbell and said, "Mrs. McCall, Timmy's been hit by a car," she ran all the way there in high heels.

———————

When I began to reconstruct my early life trauma, I realized that even when I got out of the incubator and went home, it would have been to a mother who hadn't had the opportunity to bond with me during the critical period right after childbirth. I didn't get to spend one second on her stomach, feeling its warmth, inhaling her smell, being calmed by the resonance of her heartbeat. Skin-to-skin contact is said to be crucial in mother-child bonding. We were both deprived of that. She was also recovering from her own life-threatening ordeal, so once I got home, she was probably less available to me than she might otherwise have been.

Her breasts dried up, meaning that source of human touch was also denied. As the baby book documented, my early-life diet consisted of formula feeding — a mixture of canned, evaporated cow's milk, sugar, and water. From a yogic and Ayurvedic perspective, this diet was low in prana, a far cry from mother's milk, fine-crafted through eons of evolution to meet infants' needs. The doctors at the hospital had been worried that I was sleeping so much that I wasn't taking in enough calories to survive. It's almost as if I was saying, *There's nothing worth staying awake for.*

A lack of physical affection was characteristic of our family life, as was the lack of verbal affection. I don't remember any hugs or kisses. Nobody ever said, "I love you." I introduced hugging to the family after returning from college, where I'd learned it from friends and lovers, but it didn't really take. Pop tried, but could only hug you if he was simultaneously punching you in the ribs. Tony, Ray, and I still laugh about it.

The only touch I remember is that Pop sometimes scratched my back when I was little, and he often asked me to scratch his after he got home from work. We also played a game, in which I pretended to be an "American Indian." I'd sound "Woo, woo, woo, woo! Woo, woo woo, woo!" as he pounded my back with the flat of his hand. I still remember the feel of those vibrations. Looking back, this might have been my very first chanting.

Once I started to grok how my relationship with my mother had affected me, I came to appreciate the importance of those morsels of affection I got from Pop. Ray told me when I couldn't fall asleep as an infant that Pop would rub my back until I did. Of course, I have no memory of that, but I must have been starved for that loving touch. I wonder if that experience influenced a rule I made as a young man: If you wouldn't rub my back, you couldn't be my girlfriend (though I was always happy to reciprocate).

Pop was a product of his era and of the Irish Catholic culture he grew up in — he may have been a psychologist, but he was shut down emotionally. I think that he truly loved me in a way that Mom wasn't capable of. But that's something I only figured out as an adult — his relentless criticism obscured my ability to feel his love. Knowing about the back rubs he gave me as an infant, and seeing all the care he put into filling in that baby book, I can see that even more clearly now.

When Pop was diagnosed with Alzheimer's disease, just after I finished my residency in primary care internal medicine, the first thing I did was tell him that I loved him. Up until that moment I never had — and he had never said the words to me. I just hoped he was able to take it in, and remember what I'd said, but I wasn't sure he still could.

My cat Spats, who had been my early-life love teacher and a source of ongoing affection, must have played a similar role to Pop's in keeping my heart from ossifying completely. Even that loving third grade teacher I had at the Catholic school probably made a difference. And then there was my big brother Ray.

After Ray left college, he moved home, which meant he was around all those years while I was growing up. He'd been an art history major, and while he was living with us, he joined the rock band The Shags. Beyond teaching me to ride a bike, he taught me about modern art and how to paint, which I did avidly in high school. He turned me onto music, and gave me guitar lessons. Ray was my buddy and a mentor — more like a cool uncle than a brother.

My relationship with Tony was never bad; he just wasn't that involved in my life. He'd moved out of the house when I was eight and never moved back. The four years before that, he was wrapped up in his experience at the fancy, suburban prep school, to which he'd won a scholarship.

Both of my parents were capable of empathy — at least intellectually. They could sympathize with victims of injustice. For a few years, they attended the church, St. Boniface, that was at the center of Milwaukee's vocal civil rights movement. Mom became the only white member of their gospel choir. With her permed grey hair and dark tan, I suspect she could have passed as black, at least in that context. After my parents retired to southeast Florida, she got involved with her church's efforts to help resettle Haitian immigrants, who were overwhelmingly Catholic.

But Mom, I came to believe, had a harder time empathizing with the people in front of her. That included family members and an infant whose needs she probably had difficulty deciphering. Pop didn't offer much help — he was obsessed with his work and not involved in childcare.

As I continued my psychological excavation project, I saw some things about myself that I did not like. I had always thought of myself as a good guy, one who tried to treat his romantic partners well. I had to admit, though, that I hadn't always been a great boyfriend — and I'd handled a few breakups poorly. I realized that, like Mom, I wasn't that good at empathy.

In relationships, I had confused fun, excitement, and intensity for depth. Perhaps because emotional nurturing was in such short supply in my early life, I had an unquenchable longing for attention. As a kid, I'd figured out that if I said something clever or achieved something noteworthy, I could get it, as when I held my own in that dinner-table debate with Tony. As a young man, attention — particularly sexual interest from women I considered cool and attractive — was the drug I used to feel okay about myself. But as with a pharmaceutical, over time you develop tolerance — necessitating an ever-higher dose or a new supply — so enduring satisfaction was always elusive.

My confusion about what's important caused a lot of suffering, and it affected my behavior adversely. I made a few spectacularly poor choices about which relationships to pursue. I paid the price, too. I was drawn to the fool's gold of attention and missed what is truly precious: Love. I couldn't see it, even when it was right there in front of me.

As I do my morning meditation, the only light in the room is over a framed painting of the Hindu warrior Goddess Durga. She sits sidesaddle on a tiger, most of her eight arms wielding weapons, though one hand holds a flower and another is raised, palm out, signaling *Have no fear*.

Eight years ago, I told a monk I'll call Swami Radha, who I met at an ashram in the west, that I'd been realizing how wounded I'd been as a child. The remedy, she told me, was to worship a Goddess. But not one who was "too nice," she said. She recommended Durga, a fierce embodiment of mother. Not my mother, *The* Mother. The swami gave me a Sanskrit Durga mantra and a postcard with a picture of the deity to put on my altar at home.

Later, I bought a reproduction of a different painting of the Goddess, which sits on my altar today.

To accompany the meditation that the swami prescribed, she added an emotional visualization. That's what's known in yoga as a Bhava — and this may have been the most effective element. Every time I inhaled and said the four words of the Durga mantra silently, I was to imagine the love of the Mother flooding into my heart. Each time I exhaled, I visualized that love circulating to every cell in my body. To this meditation practice, I added a hand gesture, called Hridaya (heart) Mudra, which the Swami Radha hadn't specified — crossing my hands over my heart. This mudra seemed to make emotions more accessible.

When I first tried the practice after returning to my Oakland home, it was like nothing I had ever experienced. As I inhaled the love into my heart, it felt like a balm soothing the biggest wound of my life. I've never tried heroin, but this is what I imagine it might feel like. That intensity dissipated over the first few weeks, yet I've used this sweet visualization ever since.

―――――――――――

While I was teaching at an ashram in the Bahamas, I attended a lecture with Vedic scholar Dr. David Frawley. Speaking with me afterwards, he said that "even atheists can benefit from Bhakti yoga," the yoga of devotion. He thought given my childhood situation that bhakti practices could be powerful for me. I wondered how I might do that. It occurred to me that I should give devotional singing a second chance.

Ever since I'd gotten into yoga, people had been dragging me to kirtans — group chanting in Sanskrit. Typically, a performer sits in the front of the room playing a harmonium, a small organ-like instrument. One hand fingers a mini-keyboard, while the other works the bellows. The singer chants a line and the audience repeats it, mimicking the delivery and any vocal inflections.

I did my best, but these performances always left me flat. I found them musically uninteresting. Surrounded by clapping and dancing yogis, I imagined that I was probably the only person in the room who felt that way.

I decided to see if I could change my mind by attending performances by a famous kirtan artist who was booked for three consecutive nights at the ashram. I went to all three concerts. The singer's baritone was rich, infused with emotion. You could feel his deep bhakti. But the major-chord melodies reminded me of something you might sing at camp. Every piece started slowly and was modulated up to a frenzy at the end. I did not find this exciting, especially after the first time.

On the final night, however, the artist covered the gospel tune "Jesus on the Mainline." This went straight to my heart. I had a similar reaction a month later back in Oakland when a kirtan band from New Orleans, which a friend assured me was more musically interesting than most, performed the spiritual, "I'll Fly Away."

I realized that African-American spirituals, and particularly gospel-inflected rhythm and blues, were my devotional music. (I would later amend that list to include Sufi devotional performances.) Maybe it was related to the hundreds of times I'd heard and sung "We Shall Overcome" as part of Milwaukee's civil rights movement. For years, I'd danced at home for exercise, but I started to incorporate more of this music into my playlists. I danced barefoot on the hardwood floor of my living room in Oakland, feeling the love of the Mother as I moved my body to the syncopation of Mavis Staples' pleading, percussive growls on "I'll Take You There."

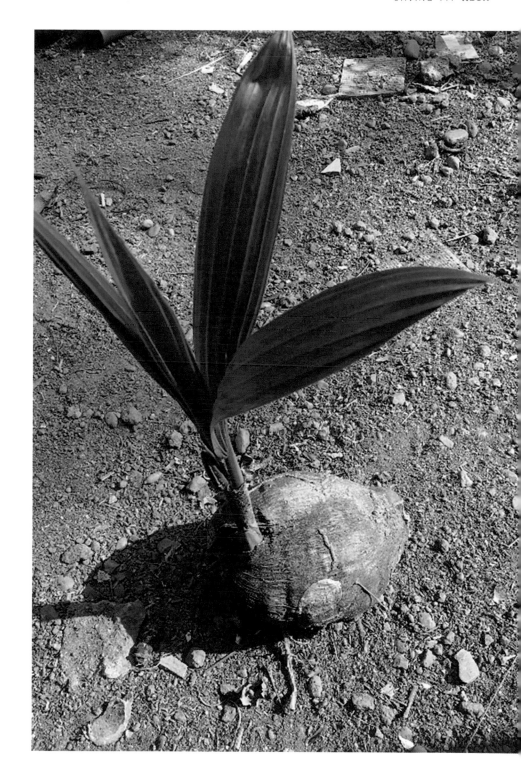

When I first figured out how badly I'd been wounded as a kid, I despaired that the damage might be irreparable. I saw that my whole life I had been blocking love from flowing out of me. Even more surprising, I realized that I'd been blocking love coming in from others. I wondered if the empathy I seemed to lack was something I could cultivate.

I knew from my training in medicine that if certain functions of the brain aren't activated early in life, the nervous system concludes that you don't need them. It sets about pruning the synapses — the connections between neurons — that make those functions possible. For example, if you don't hear Japanese phonemes by 18 months of age, it's said, you'll never learn to speak like a native. I wasn't sure I'd be able to learn the language of love.

But I had seen yoga and Ayurveda make a huge difference in my spine, in my chronic muscle tension, and in my ability to sleep, so I had faith that they could help me in other ways too. Faith in yoga, it needs to be said, is different from faith as it's thought of in religion. It's not about accepting anything blindly, as in an article of faith. Rather as you walk the yogic path and watch it unfold, you see that it works — and that experience gives you faith. With persistence, and the right tools, I thought I might be able to grow the emotional muscles that I either lacked entirely or had never exercised.

So every morning, to this day, I chant mantras and pray to a Goddess whom I don't believe ever existed — at least, not outside of people's imaginations. By cultivating the feeling of bonding with the Mother, however, I am attempting to tap into the neuroplasticity that I hope will enable me to rewire my emotional brain. I think it's working.

Despite their anti-war stance and involvement in civil rights, my parents were less enlightened when it came to homosexuality. One Christmas while I was in college, I gave Mom a book that came highly recommended from a knowledgeable friend who worked at a feminist bookstore in Madison. It was called *Of Woman Born*, written by the poet Adrienne Rich. The next time I returned home for a visit, my mother was spitting mad. "She practically admits that she's a homosexual," Mom said. Imagine that.

When I look back, I wonder if perhaps the book hit too close to home. The book is a feminist analysis of how the institution of motherhood was shaped by the patriarchy. Growing up in a conservative Irish Catholic household, Mom must have felt that marriage and motherhood were her only options. With her fierce independence, I couldn't have seen her lasting more than a week in a convent. She'd trained as a schoolteacher — that and nursing being the only professions available to young women like her — but as expected she gave that up when she married Pop. Her never-ending projects may have been more interesting and compelling to her than raising children. She was a woman of enormous talent. Perhaps being a mother was not what she was meant to do. Had that possibility existed then, I think she could have been a formidable CEO.

But in recent years I've had another thought, one which seems to fit the facts. Could my mother have been a suppressed lesbian? If that was true, to survive her strict Catholic upbringing, she might have had to wall off those feelings so far from her awareness that even she wouldn't have even known they were there. I sometimes even wonder whether my mannish Mom, had she been born in a different age, might have transitioned to a male identity.

Pop once told me he didn't think there was any way to be homosexual *and* happy. Aberrant sexual behavior was a major focus of his psychological work. In his textbook, *The Varieties of Abnormality*, his assessment of homosexuality was unsparing, appearing right before the section on pedophilia. He saw it as pathological. He refused to use the word gay in conversation, grousing that a perfectly good term to express cheerfulness had been hijacked, but he never used demeaning names.

While both my parents were critical of homosexuality, they also seemed to be unusually interested in it. At the dinner table at the lake house, they regularly discussed the "femme/butch" couples at the country club — my parents' term for masculine women married to effeminate men. Although he never said anything to me, I suspect Pop was petrified that I would turn out to be gay. Maybe that in part explains why he seemed so obsessed with my long hair. When I was 12, two of my friends told me he'd approached them to ask if I liked girls. "Of course," they told him.

For years, Pop consulted at the largest maximum-security prison in Wisconsin. Once when I was 18, I accompanied him there, posing as his student. One charming psychopath whom he interviewed detailed his sex life in prison. "He's not a homosexual," Pop told me afterwards. It's just that if he wants to have sex, men were his only option. Years later, as I came to wonder about my father's sexuality, too, I reflected back on this conversation. I thought to myself, *And how long were you off in the Navy during World War II, Pop?*

———————

To try to boost the effectiveness of the heart opening practice I began in 2010, a few years ago I added one more yogic tool: intention. A yogic intention, also known as a *sankalpa*, is like an affirmation, but it's more about what you are going to do, and less about what you hope will happen as a result. So, "I am practicing yoga every morning" is a sankalpa. "I am going to lose 30 pounds by beach season," is a desire, not a sankalpa. Based on that desire, however, you might develop a sankalpa, for example, to get more exercise or fast one day per week.

The idea of a sankalpa is that you come up with a statement, a promise you make to yourself. It may not be true at the moment, but it's something you hope to bring into being. By repeating it again and again verbatim, you implant it in your subconscious — and in your neural circuitry. The sankalpa I developed embodied everything I felt I had missed as a child: *I am feeling loved, protected, nourished and cherished by the Mother*. I recite it every morning and evening, right before my meditation practice. I've paired this sankalpa with my mantra, first saying one then the other repeatedly, as I look at the picture of Durga on my altar. Closing my eyes, I can still see that image of the Goddess in my mind, as I begin to focus on my mantra and the feeling of being bathed in love.

I used to joke that Theresa, a nurse I met at a government clinic where I was working in the years just after residency, was my surrogate mom. If so, she was definitely the warm, terry cloth version. Theresa laughed a lot — at jokes, at people's stories, at the craziness of life, and at the stupidity of the bureaucrats who oversaw our work.

In many ways we were as different as could be. She was decades my senior and a devout Catholic. Hers was not the rigid Catholicism of my childhood, though, but a more loving, compassionate, joyful version. Perhaps I would still be a believer if I'd met more people like her as a kid.

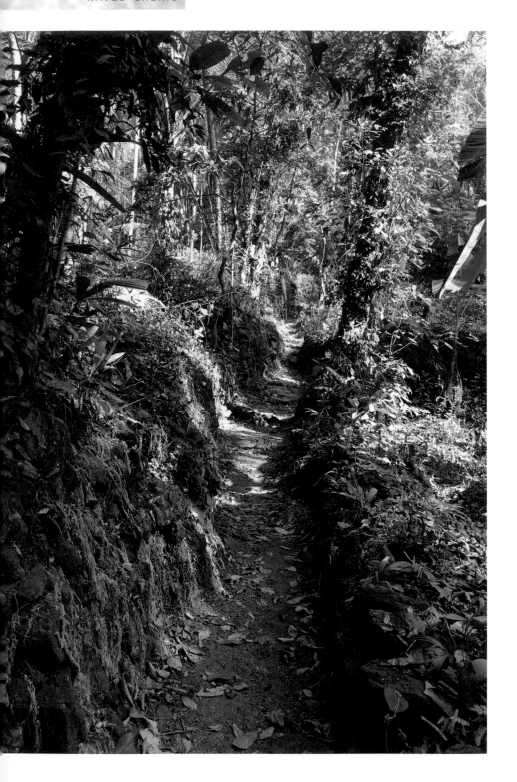

I attended Christmas dinners at her house and they were far more formal than anything I'd experienced at our family table, or would have chosen on my own. Everyone wore their Sunday best. The multi-course meals were served on her finest china. But they were huge amounts of fun. I reveled in her, her family, and the obvious love between them all. When her grandchildren started arriving, she became obsessed with them, so different from what I'd seen with Mom. It occurred to me that I had missed out on grandmotherly love completely: Pop's parents died before he got married; Mom's parents died when I was a toddler, and from the sound it, they wouldn't have taken much interest in me anyway.

When I was trying to reprogram my calcified heart, I would imagine Theresa and how she lit up with joy when she discussed her latest grandchild, also named Timothy. I thought, too, about the fierce love my friend Linda had for her two sons, including the one born in the bedroom of my Burlington home. Imagining those relationships as I recited my Durga mantra brought me a visceral sensation of the motherly love I'd missed out on.

In my family, emotions like sadness, fear, and shame were never spoken of, but anger was given full expression. Directly by my mother, and mostly indirectly by my father — as with his endless criticism and his looking for a fight when he came home in a bad mood. Starting in the seventh grade, I channeled my own anger, along with my idealism, into protesting the Vietnam War in the surprisingly lively streets of Milwaukee during the late 1960s. This was my next major exposure to chanting: "Ho Ho Ho Chi Mihn, the NLF is gonna win." "Whadda we want? Peace! When do we want it? Now!"

Around the turn of the millennium, I was part of a group of health care activists among whom anger at the status quo was endemic. I was the executive director, and one of the many co-founders, of a group of health care professionals who collected signatures and got a binding ballot initiative to bring universal health care to the State of Massachusetts. The effort — which came five years before future Governor Mitt Romney enacted such a plan — nearly succeeded.

However, as I continued my personal psychological exploration, I reached the conclusion that while I was good at righteous indignation, righteous indignation wasn't good for me. I'd grown up in a household steeped in anger, and I found myself wanting to move beyond it. The more I practiced yoga, the more I saw how angry and dysfunctional the health care activism scene could be.

Just as I made the decision to leave activism behind, I concluded that a lot of it was futile anyway. I watched a pair of brilliant physicians, professors at a local medical school who were part of the movement, fail to convince people of their positions — not because they didn't make sense, but because audiences could feel their anger and were turned off.

The next morning, I woke with an epiphany: You can't change the world by arguing better. Or at least I couldn't.

———————

Many depictions of Durga, including the first one Swami Radha gave me, show her riding a lion. From the beginning, though, I felt drawn to images I found of the Goddess atop a tiger. Years later I told this to the swami. She thought it was because the tiger is sweeter than the lion. Perhaps, I thought, I was connecting to the same feline energy with the tiger that I'd experienced with my childhood pet Spats.

Soon after I began to chant the Durga mantra, female cats starting coming into my life. Two different neighborhood cats on different occasions jumped in an open window of my Oakland apartment to visit. The same thing happened while I was teaching in Austria. One pre-dawn morning at home, my neighbor's cat hopped in and curled up in my lap as I silently recited my mantra.

These cats were different from the male cats I'd been around. They weren't interested in being petted per se. They were looking for love, not just physical sensation. If you stroked them absent-mindedly, which was always fine with the cats I'd known, they quickly grew bored and left. They wanted you to watch them, talk to them, relate to them.

———————

Less than three months after finishing cancer treatment, I notice that my meditation is less focused. As I sit on the cushion in my yoga room in Vermont, my mind flits from one thought to another: Planning my day, memories of a woman I knew in college — everything, it seems, but staying with my mantra.

To try to open my wounded heart and access my shutdown emotions, seven years earlier I had placed my meditation focus at the heart center. The heart focus was a good decision. It deepened the sensation that the love of the Mother was flowing into me. That helped me to re-pattern the dysfunctional emotional habits that got me through a difficult childhood, but which no longer served me.

But my gut tells me it is time for a change. Yoga teaches that when the focus in meditation is in the heart, emotions flow freely — but so do thoughts. I have made huge progress in healing my emotional wounding, which I hope will continue. But now I decide to lower the focus during meditation to the navel center, the chakra called Manipura, Sanskrit for "city of jewels."

That, the tradition teaches, tends to be more grounding than when you place your meditative focus in either the heart center or the third eye — the two other most commonly used chakras for meditation. Yogis believe that meditating at the Manipura chakra facilitates healing, and God knows I'm in need of that. The next morning, as I bring my awareness down to the area along the spine at the level of the navel, I immediately notice a difference. I feel more grounded. My mind still wanders, but not nearly as much.

———————

When I was looking to heal my wounded heart, a Sanskrit mantra and an image of an Indian Goddess came to my aid. The Virgin Mother and the Hail Mary prayer that I mouthed thousands of times as a child — my fingers navigating the plastic beads on the baby blue rosary I was given for my First Communion — might work just as well for some. But given my history with the Church, these were too fraught for me to use. Yoga does not belong only to Hinduism. It's a philosophy and a practice that can go with any religion, or with none.

To this day, I count my mantras using mala beads, a necklace made of 108 seeds of the Indian Rudraksha tree, strung on a loop. This isn't as far from my roots as it might seem. In the Middle Ages, Muslim traders sold Indian prayer beads to Crusaders who brought them home, where they became the first rosaries.

In an unexpected way, my experiences with Hinduism have brought me closer to the religion of my childhood.

As I see it, Christ, who fasted, meditated, and preached universal love, lived like a yogi. And my own lifestyle is not so different from that of my cousin, who was a Benedictine monk.

One of the family treasures I unearthed going through the Vermont lake house before it sold was a reproduction of Raphael's Italian Renaissance portrait of Madonna and Child, with a beatific St. John the Baptist looking on. The small round image, which belonged to my mother, is mounted in an ornate golden wood frame, with one small corner now chipped off.

In Raphael's depiction, Mary has classic pitta facial features: an angular nose, rosy cheeks and lips, and deep-set eyes full of tejas (TAY-juss), the power of discernment and clear-seeing that yogis value. That image of the Christ child in his mother's arms now sits in the room where I meditate each morning. It's right next to a statue of Ganesha, the elephant-headed remover of obstacles, who is balanced on his forearms in a yoga pose.

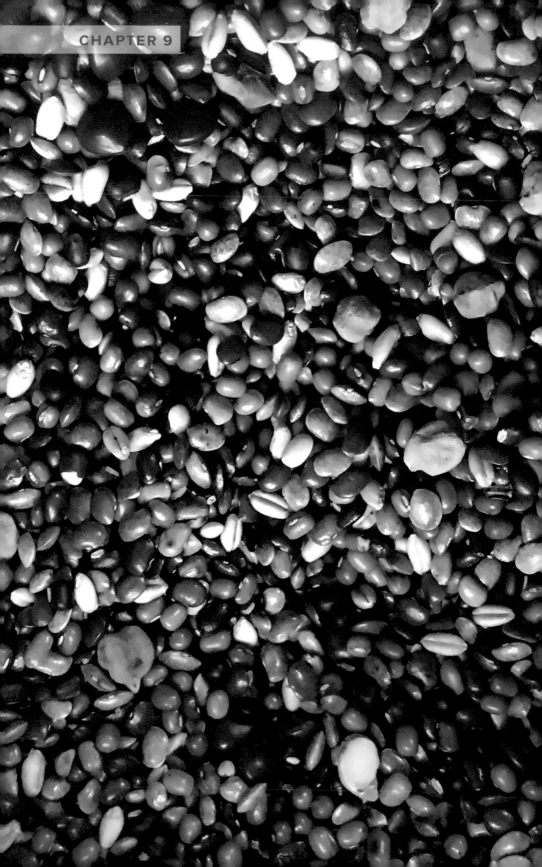

CHAPTER 9

"If you want a long life – which is the means for achieving Dharma (life purpose), Artha (material and physical well-being) and Sukha (happiness) – put your faith in the teachings of Ayurveda."

— Vagbhata

SCIENCE OF LIFE

It's the evening of my first day back in Kerala. I'm here for more Ayurvedic treatments — still trying to recover from the ravages of chemoradiation, which I finished eight months ago. Krishna's 18-year-old daughter Aiswarya holds her father's phone up for the younger kids, gathered around her on the front porch. Laughter cascades. On the screen is a close-up of Donald Trump, taken from his State of the Union speech, remixed to show him lip-synching the song *Despacito*. Seated behind him, the Vice President and the Speaker of the House bob their heads left and right in sync with the Latin beat.

Smart phones are spreading fast in India, and children are getting exposed to foreign media and culture like never before. These kids have grown up loving the music of popular films, Bollywood ones in Hindi and Mollywood ones in Malayalam. When I was here a year ago, they had never seen a western music video; now they can't live without them.

Aiswarya asks me a question but her accent is so thick that I can't make out what she's saying. Although

English was taught at her school, the students don't learn it as well as middle class kids in the many private schools where only English is used. She says it again and this time I get it: JOO-stun BEE-bah. Justin Bieber. I tell her that in America, his fans call themselves Beliebers.

"I am not a fan," she informs me. "I just like some of his songs."

———

Ayurveda, India's ancient system of holistic medicine, includes a wide range of treatments including herbs, oil massages, and, in ancient times, even rhinoplasties (nose jobs) to repair damage inflicted in war or accidents. Today, the 6th century BCE surgeon Sushruta, author of one of the major Ayurvedic texts, is considered the "father of plastic surgery." When the British arrived in the early 1600s, their doctors had never seen anything like Ayurveda's advanced surgical techniques.

Yet the British almost succeeded in killing Ayurveda. The East India Company, the British private trading corporation that controlled India for hundreds of years, closed all Ayurvedic medical colleges in 1833 and banned the practice. Over the coming generations, as masters died and weren't replaced, much knowledge was lost.

Though a revival of Ayurvedic medicine began in the late 19th century, as part of the growing Indian nationalist movement, Ayurvedic colleges weren't officially reopened until India gained independence in 1947. Thus, most of what is now taught in Indian Ayurvedic medical colleges could be called "reconstituted" Ayurveda. There are no living masters who can answer such questions as the identity of many herbs described in the ancient manuscripts, or how to make some medicines, so scholars and researchers pore through Ayurvedic texts and try to figure out what was being indicated. Often, the answers will never be known.

In Kerala, and some other areas of India, Ayurveda survived in the underground. Chandukutty got a full download from his father and grandfather, who in turn had learned it from theirs, starting young. At the age of four, Chandukutty began to learn the family's secret massage techniques by massaging his father, an exacting master, every day. As a boy, he helped locate the medicines in the wild, cut and prepared them and cooked the various oils. He learned to chant mantras in Sanskrit from the Malabar-area's preferred Ayurvedic text, Vagbhata's *Ashtanga Hridiyam*, etched onto palm leaves.

While herbal medicines and the intense detoxification regimen known as pancha karma get most of the press, the foundation of Ayurveda's approach is dietary and lifestyle advice. I should mention here that in the three Ayurvedic centers I've visited in Kerala, no one has ever talked about pancha karma. Vaidyars in the Malabar-region of Kerala like Chandukutty treat health conditions successfully using other techniques.

I've come to rely on Ayurveda in managing my own health and it informs the yoga therapy work I do. But it was not always that way. Although I was aware in the late 1990s that many yoga therapists incorporated Ayurveda into their work, I was skeptical. With its talk of bodily humors and the "elements" of earth, water, fire and air and space, and its emphasis on the health effects of different seasons and climates, it reminded me of ancient Greek medicine. Despite our reverence for Hippocrates as the "father of modern scientific medicine," I'd learned in school that the healing system he practiced was quaint, ancient nonsense. When I started writing my book, *Yoga as Medicine* in the year 2000, I decided to leave Ayurveda out.

But as yogis like to say, the universe had other plans for me. Starting in the fall of 2004, I became a scholar-in-residence at the Kripalu Center for Yoga and Health, in the Berkshire mountains of western Massachusetts. It was there that I completed the first draft of the book. I lived in a small house, which at one time had housed the guru, located a few hundred yards up in the woods from the main building.

My housemate, Swami Shivananda, was an itinerant Dutch musician turned yogi and Ayurvedic practitioner. With his long, white beard and red face, he looked like a 19th century poster of Kris Kringle. The only difference was that instead of a wearing a red suit, this Hindu monk wore orange. Swamiji, as we called him, was teaching in Kripalu's new Ayurveda training program. Drinking tea in the shared kitchen between our respective living quarters on the first floor of the house, we regularly discussed yoga and Ayurveda.

One day, he offered to do an Ayurvedic assessment of my pulse. He placed three fingers on my right wrist, and spent a couple of minutes tuning into the sensations with his fingertips. He said he noted an elevated level of vata dosha.

According to Ayurvedic theory, a multitude of factors in my recent experience made a vata elevation likely: I had been toiling for months to meet my book deadline; it was getting cold, winds gusting erratically in the Berkshires as October turned to November; I had just moved out of Boston, where I'd lived for years; and then spent a couple of months at the uninsulated lakc house in Vermont, which could be an icebox on fall mornings.

Vata is associated with certain properties including

coldness, roughness, irregularity, movement, change-ability, and excessive mental activity. As I was later to figure out, I've likely had vata derangement since birth — and the circumstances of that period in my life would no doubt have intensified it. Given how stressful the pregnancy was — and how afraid and unhappily pregnant my mother was — I suspect my vata may have even been out of whack even before I was born.

The antidote Swamiji suggested was to adopt a more regular schedule of eating and sleeping. He recommended that I consume warm, well-cooked, unctuous meals — that is, foods cooked with an abundance of healthy fats like ghee. I also followed his advice, and booked an Ayurvedic massage with heated oil. These suggestions embodied the Ayurvedic principle of using opposite properties to correct imbalances: in this case, warmth, smoothness, regularity, and unctuousness. I followed his advice and within a few days I was sleeping better, my concentration had improved, and I felt more grounded in my body. The longer I followed his advice, the deeper the benefits seemed to become. This helped me with my work on the book — and led to a change of heart about including a discussion of Ayurveda in it.

A few weeks after Swami Shivananda first took my pulse, I received an email from my friend Josh, who had just graduated from acupuncture school in Boston. He was hoping that I would write a blurb promoting his new private practice. I told him that since I'd never sampled his work, I would only write a blurb if he drove to Kripalu and gave me a couple of treatments. Soon he visited for a weekend.

Before Josh arrived, Swamiji again took my pulse. He found that I still had a vata imbalance, though improved. Using a different system of pulse diagnosis that he'd learned in acupuncture school, Josh diagnosed me as having a *kidney jing* deficiency — which I was told was in some ways analogous to excess vata, as Ayurveda conceptualizes it.

Josh treated me once on Saturday and again Sunday morning with electroacupuncture, in which a small electric current is passed through acupuncture needles. After these two treatments, I felt relaxed and centered. When Swamiji took my pulse again, he discovered my vata imbalance had greatly improved.

Once again, as had happened when I was studying with Patricia and being treated by Hiroyuki, it occurred to me that two ancient holistic systems, in this case Ayurveda and traditional Chinese medicine (TCM), were seeing the

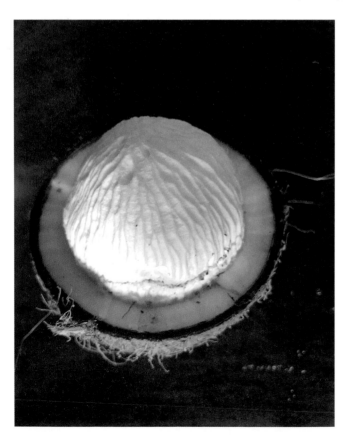

same imbalances. They just used different metaphors to describe them, and had different therapeutic strategies. But whether you call the energetic flow in the body that both systems apprehend "prana" or "chi," they are talking about the same, very real, phenomenon. And to experts in these fields, its manifestations in the body are observable via the pulse and other methods — even if modern medicine hasn't found a way to measure them yet.

It is Thanksgiving in the US. This is the earliest I've been to Kerala in the winter season. Everything is verdant, wetter than I've ever seen here. There is light rain and it's overcast most days, though the sun breaks through and, in those moments, it can feel hot. By local standards evenings are cool, yet I sleep covered by a single sheet, wearing only shorts.

Today is the first day of the three-month Ayurvedic treatment program that Krishna had mapped out for me when I told him I'd been invited to give the keynote address at a big conference in the UK. These treatments are designed to help me recover from the chemoradiation and to prepare me for the trip to England.

But because he doesn't want to tax my body too much, Krishna is planning many rest days interspersed with active treatment days. The plan we agreed to calls for a total of 42 days of treatment, interspersed with 36 days of rest, and another 21 days of rest at the end. After that, I should be sufficiently restored to be able to fly to London to give my speech and teach a couple of workshops. This will be the longest Ayurvedic treatment I've ever had, and I am looking forward to it.

Krishna tells me he's worried that the treatments he's planning might encourage growth in any lingering cancer cells in my body. I suspect he's remembering Chandukutty's warning from last year.

"You know what Krishna?" I say. "Last time I got treatment from you, my tonsil and lymph nodes got smaller. I don't think it's going to make the cancer stronger. The treatment doesn't fight the cancer. I do. It makes me stronger and more balanced, and better able to fight. Let's do the full treatment."

This pours out of me, and instantly, we both know it's correct.

"I don't know where that came from," I say. "Maybe from God."

Krishna looks toward the ceiling "Yes, he says, "that came from the God." It may have also come from my growing confidence in shaping the course of my Ayurvedic treatments. If Chandukutty were still alive, I would have deferred to him. But I feel going forward that Krishna and I can work in a more collaborative fashion.

Today we begin with Dhanya Kizhi, that is, dry poultice therapy. As I lie face up on the wood table, Krishna warms a collection of seeds and grains in a clay pot, stirring it with a wood spatula. The only compromise with modernity is the gas flame from a propane tank with which he heats the mixture. Once he deems it sufficiently hot, he transfers the seeds to a muslin bag, which he uses to stroke my body. After perhaps ten minutes, when the bag cools to warm, he opens it up over the clay pot and reheats the mixture.

As he moves the bag back and forth over each part of my body, its shifting contents make a sound that resembles a maraca. The only areas he skips are the genitals and the head — which Ayurveda believes should never be heated. The ingredients are all edible: wheat, horse gram and a round, reddish-colored seed that Krishna doesn't know the English for, which he tells me is particularly helpful for joint pain in rheumatoid arthritis patients.

After half an hour, he has me turn to lie on my stomach and applies oil to my back. It's familiar to me from treatments in prior years: camphor dissolved into coconut oil. The smell is pungent, almost like turpentine. I find it deeply relaxing. He massages the back of my body and after I turn over again, the front. He stands at the head of the table and leans way over me delivering long strokes with both arms simultaneously, from my hands to my shoulders, looping down the sides of the chest and abdomen, then back up the middle in repeated loops.

I've established a morning routine in Kerala that resembles what I do at home. I wake at 4:30 a.m. and take my Ayurvedic pulse for a few minutes as I lie in bed. It's said this is the very best time to assess the pulse, before it responds to the hustle and bustle of the day.

Another part of my morning ritual is an examination of my tongue in the mirror. It's one of the best ways, besides pulse, to detect Ayurvedic imbalances. As I inspect my tongue, I look to see if there is an abnormal coating. That would signal a buildup of toxicity, known as ama (AH-muh). A thin white coating is considered normal. Today, a few days after my arrival in India, there's no abnormal coating, though there had been before I got here.

The cracks in the tongue that had turned up during my vata-deranging last few weeks in the States — as I traveled out of town to teach and prepared for this long trip — have also disappeared. The surface looks smooth. And I no longer see any fasciculations, those bag-of-worms movements the tongue sometimes makes even when you try to still it. Nor are there any furrows on the surface of the tongue. These are both signs of elevated vata. Just a few days of treatments, and all these signs of imbalance are gone.

I scrape my tongue with a U-shaped copper implement. Starting at the back, I draw its broad surface forward toward the tip a few times. Then I brush my teeth. Next, I place warm water and a pinch of salt in a neti pot, also made of copper, which has a narrow spout on one side. Leaning over the sink, my head turned to one side, I tip the pot and the soothing warm saline runs to the back of one nostril, turns the corner at the back of the throat, and exits through the other nostril. I breathe though my mouth as I do this. I repeat this a few times for each nostril and I'm done.

Tongue scraping is part of the morning ritual recommended in Ayurveda. Scraping the tongue is said to remove some toxicity from the body. Similarly, cleaning the nasal passages, which comes from the world of yoga, removes mucus, pollen, inflammatory cells and particulate matter that's settled in the nose, and has been shown to improve sinus health.

After washing my face, and drinking a container of warm water, I return to my room to begin my morning practice. I open the windows to bring in the cool morning air. My preference would be to leave them open all night but because of mosquitoes and the maniacal barking of neighborhood dogs in the wee hours, I've stopped doing this. I turn on the little light I've mounted over the makeshift altar I've created in my room, consisting of a framed painting of the warrior Goddess Durga, weapons perched in many of her eight arms. In front of her stands a small brass statue of Ganesha, the elephant-headed Hindu deity.

I do 30–45 minutes of asana. This is followed by chanting, pranayama, and meditation, which take a little over an hour. While I sit in meditation, I often hear from down-stairs PSSSSSSSSSSS Ttthh, PSSSSSSSSSSS Ttthh, the sound of steam building up and releasing from the cook-ing of the ragi puttu, which will be my breakfast. Ragi is a rich-tasting traditional pumpernickel-brown grain, increasingly difficult to find here. Puttu are steam cakes with alternating, hockey-puck-sized layers of grain and thinner layers of coconut. Topped with curry, and some-times tiny, sweet bananas, it is scrumptious.

———————

Two weeks into this trip, based on my pulse checks and my examination of my tongue, my vata comes into balance. I suspect it's normal for the first time in my life. I started checking my Ayurvedic pulse regularly in 2005. Since then I've had a vata imbalance that has never gone away — regardless of the season of year, the time of day, or whatever else was going on. Sometimes the imbalance has been less than at other times, but it's never disap-peared. This change to me is a sign that everything I've been doing is paying off. I feel great — and the pulse is showing that I should.

Also noticeable is how much faster my body is re-sponding to Krishna's work. I've had the treatments he's giving me before and have never had tight areas open so quickly. It occurs to me that this is likely due to the syn-ergy between the myofascial release (MFR) work Ginny did last summer and the Ayurvedic massage techniques that Krishna is using. The latter are based on marma points — the junctions where energy lines, or nadis, come together. This is something Krishna learned from Chan-dukutty as a way of opening up energetic blockages.

Chandukutty's study of the martial art of Kalaripay-attu taught him about marma points and influenced his practice of Ayurveda. Marma points comprise 108 locations on the body, and Kalari practitioners learned which of these to target in battle. Blows to one marma would cause instant death to their opponents, to another point a loss of consciousness, to a third an inability to move for several hours, and so on. Such effects were due to the way the flow of prana was blocked.

When their own warriors were injured in battle, Kalari masters figured out over the years how to use certain massage techniques aimed at the marma points to undo the blockages, and restore the flow of pranic energy. These principles of marma therapy made their way into Kerala-style Ayurveda. A number of Kalari masters to this day are expert in treating fractures, dislocations, and other injuries.

One day early in my stay, I take a walk after breakfast. As I cross the elevated stone and cement walkway that runs alongside the paddy, I turn right at the road. Feeling energetic, I walk farther than I have so far this trip. Near a major intersection, I spot a temple that Krishna had taken me to once or twice on prior trips. I walk past the outdoor pool, where worshipers can bathe before entering the temple, though few seem to use it. At the entrance, I add my flip-flops to the large collection of shoes on either side of the dirt path.

I'm dressed in shorts, not the dhoti that Krishna would normally lend me if I were going to a temple. Worse, I walk in forgetting to remove my shirt. The Vedic priest who recognizes me from past years pantomimes taking his shirt off. After the second time, I realize what he's indicating.

The temple has a powerful shakti — energy in Sanskrit — which I can feel as soon as I enter. My legs feel more solidly grounded. I visit the idol in an enclosed shrine in the middle of the open-air inner courtyard. It's not a deity that is familiar to me. I walk in a clockwise direction, as I've been taught, circumambulating the building inside and out.

As I walk outside, an older man in a dhoti peers from an open door and beckons me over. Because he can see that I'm a visitor who probably doesn't know much about the place, he wants to explain to me that the Deva of this temple — its god — is Mahasudarshana, which means "great vision." That's the idol I'd seen in the courtyard. Later I would learn that the deity is one of the less well-known avatars of Vishnu.

When I first arrived at Krishna's, I noticed a small lamp-black cat and her two tiny kittens, one also black, the other a tiger cat. The three cats were always together when I saw them in the yard. When the kittens wander too far, the mother softly mews, not intermittently as every other cat I've ever seen does, but continuously, for minutes at a time, until they return.

This morning as I am putting on my flip-flops out front, the tiger kitten is perched on the resin chair next to the porch. I look at it from several feet away and meow. It looks back at me, sweetly, its eyelids getting heavy — but I know better than to approach. Bindu had tried that with the black kitten soon after I arrived, and was rewarded with scratches and bite marks on the back of her hand. Although cats are abundant here, none are kept as pets. They are wary of humans. If you get too close, they bolt.

The black kitten, which Aiswarya named Litu, shares more than fur color with its mother. It often mews continuously, for no apparent reason. Whether it's nature or nurture, this kitten seems to have followed in its mother's footsteps as a singer. As I sit on the treatment table this morning, I hear faintly the tell-tale non-stop cry from one, or perhaps both, of these cats. I point out the sound to Krishna, who is waiting a few more minutes before he wipes the oil from my body, before sending me off to bathe. I tell him we should rename the serenading black kitten Justin Bieber.

———————

It amazes me that Krishna rides Manoj's new motorcycle every day, while Manoj uses his old one, which some mornings doesn't start. When I was here late last year, he'd just bought the bike after having saved for five years to buy it. I assume that he judges that his brother needs a reliable bike for his work more than he does.

"Are other families around here like this?" I ask Krishna. You don't see this kind of selfless sharing among siblings in America — and I certainly didn't see it in my own family.

"Very rare," he says. "Around here they are having many problems." He says that he and Manoj "have always shared everything, based on needs."

They don't have a functioning television. They never go out to restaurants or the movies. There's no fancy anything anywhere.

They are the happiest family I've ever seen.

———————

Another day, Krishna's nephews Appu, 11, and his older brother Kanaan, 15, are playing soccer in the front yard. On each end of the 20-yard field, plastic buckets mark the goals. They contest possession but seem to make very few goals. Each time the ball escapes, one of them has to run down the sloping hill toward the paddy. Finally, Kanaan scores on a breakaway. There is no celebration, and no evidence that anyone is keeping score. Seconds later they are contesting the ball again. It took Tony and me a long time to figure out that not keeping score on the tennis court was the key to making it fun again.

On my way home from the temple today, I pass a lone cow in the middle of a field. This is a well-fed animal, not like the every-rib-visible ones I've often seen in this country. She moos repeatedly, a single baritone diphthong.

The first summers of my life were spent in a home that my parents converted from a one-room schoolhouse in Vermont. Out the back door was Farmer Young's pasture. I remember on summer days, when I was probably about four, climbing through the fence to wander among his cows, brown ones and black-and-white Holsteins. My mother, distracted by her thoughts or some home improvement project, probably had no idea I'd left the house.

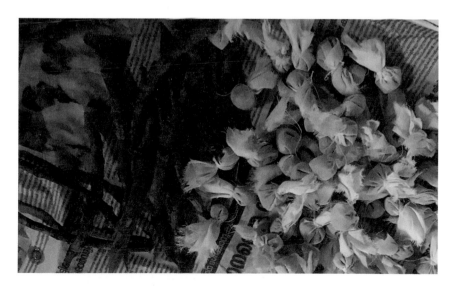

I'd squish my toes in cow pies, so cool and refreshing on summer afternoons during hot spells. Their manure wasn't sticky and didn't have much smell. It was just well-digested hay and whatever clover or Timothy grass they ate. Ayurveda believes your digestive fire, known as agni (Ugg-nee), is healthy when it turns your food to the equivalent of cleanly-burnt ash.

As I pass by, I do my best to imitate her call. I got a lot of practice as a kid. Oooooahhhh. She looks over at me. I moo again. Oooooahhhh. She returns the greeting. Turning only her head, she continues to track me as I round the bend and move away from her. I'm guessing she hasn't heard much mooing from humans before.

————————————

As I scoop ghee onto my lunch, Aiswarya tells me that I'm eating too much saturated fat. She's taking a year-long science review course to prepare her for the ultra-competitive national exam, hoping to secure a place in an Ayurvedic medical college. That's where she heard that you should avoid these fats.

For decades, physicians and nutritionists believed that dietary fat was a major culprit in heart disease and recommended that everyone should avoid it as much as possible. But recent research has questioned that notion. Such saturated fats as those in olive oil and pasture-raised cow's milk appear to be heart healthy for most people. And the low-fat and non-fat foods that were recommended in their place — which were often high in low-quality carbohydrates — appear to have fueled the epidemics of obesity and Type 2 diabetes affecting adults and children worldwide. The same happened in India, too: It has been dubbed the "diabetes capital of the world," with an estimated 72 million cases in 2017. That number is expected to increase to 134 million by the year 2025.

Ghee, especially this ghee, I tell Aiswarya, is medicine for me. A retiree Krishna knows makes it from the milk of his two, well-loved cows. According to Ayurveda, ghee is the only fat that increases the agni, aiding digestion, and yet it doesn't inflame pitta. "With my tendency toward vata derangement, this is exactly what I need," I say. Ayurveda views clarified butter as the essence of the love of the cow, a healthy fat that makes its way to every tissue so effectively that it is often used as a vehicle to deliver herbs to remote areas of the body.

I am adding ghee to my meals and munching a handful of nuts in my room before I come down to eat because the high-fat content slows the absorption of sugar and starches from the diet. Slower absorption means a lower spike in blood sugar and lower levels of insulin, both of which may fuel cancer. Because ghee contains no animal protein, which also may fuel cancer, it's better than butter. And this ghee makes every meal, already delicious, taste even better.

———————

Finding resonance with the metabolic theory of cancer, which I've been reading about since I got back to India, I plan to eat fewer carbohydrates. I quickly realize, however, that this is not going to be possible in Krishna's home. The vegetarian food the family eats and that I share is mostly carbohydrates. I have asked to not have any white rice or potatoes, which the body quickly turns to sugar, but carbs still dominate.

But this is beautiful freshly cooked food, often organic and local, and always prepared with love. This was the food I was eating a year ago, when my tonsil and lymph nodes both became noticeably smaller, so I don't think the carbs could have been doing that much harm.

However, Bindu is continually asking me if I would like another serving of food, and trying to put more rice on my plate, which I am always declining. In my experience, many Indian hosts get great satisfaction when you eat large portions, so I worry that Bindu thinks I turn down her offers because I don't appreciate her food. That's not the case — her meals are fabulous. But listening to my body, I know that the amounts of food she keeps offering are more than what I should be eating.

But I feel bad for Bindu. So, one night, when she appears at my door with a slice of watermelon about 90 minutes after dinner, I accept it and thank her. I know that according to Ayurveda, melon combines poorly with other foods — and if eaten so close to a meal could lead to indigestion. Although it's not as sweet as the watermelon I'm used to back home, it tastes good, and I don't notice any problems in the short term. In the middle of the night, however, I get up to go to the bathroom and can taste the spicy onion, tomato, and garbanzo bean curry from dinner.

Ayurveda likens digestion to cooking. Imagine you're browning onions, and you need to keep cooking them for several more minutes in order to caramelize them. If you add watery vegetables before this happens, though, the onions will never caramelize. And that's what the watermelon did to the contents of my stomach. They didn't cook right. I decided that I won't be making that mistake again.

During the three days that Chandukutty stayed at the house after he was discharged from the hospital last year, I got to ask him a few questions. One concerned something I'd wondered about for a long time — my constitution, or prakriti, as it's known in Sanskrit. Over the years, a few Ayurvedic practitioners in the West had told me I am a pitta-vata, which I accepted. My lean frame and sharp features certainly look like a combination of these two doshas.

But I'd been thinking that I had a watery, loving kapha side, too, which — for reasons related to my traumatic start in life, and the lack of maternal bonding — didn't develop as much as it might have. Based on the pulse diagnosis I did in bed every morning, I'd come to believe that I might be tridoshic, the rarest constitution.

"What's my prakriti, Vaidyar?" I asked Chandukutty one day. He made no effort to reach for my wrist. Although he often performed a brief pulse examination with new patients, I came to believe that was just a dog and pony show — because they expected him to do something to evaluate them. It didn't tell him anything he hadn't already known.

"Tridoshic," he said.

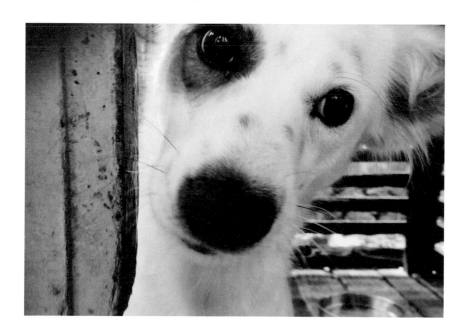

A lot of people are skeptical of typing systems like Ayurveda, as I had been, but recent scientific evidence suggests that there is a genetic basis for the differences between vatas, pittas, and kaphas. Researchers at the Institute of Genomics and Integrative Biology (IGIB) in Delhi studied subjects whose inborn constitution was judged by two Ayurvedic physicians as either predominantly vata, pitta or kapha — in other words, the more common mixed types were excluded.

Testing revealed differences in both genes and blood test results that are consistent with the Ayurvedic understanding of doshas. Kaphas had significantly higher levels of blood cholesterol and triglycerides, lower levels of "good" HDL cholesterol, and showed up-regulation of genes involved in cell building. Pittas had higher blood counts and over-expression of genes associated with immunity. Vatas had more genes associated with enzyme activity and intracellular transport.

In another study, researchers from the University of Pune found genetic evidence that pittas are more likely to be fast metabolizers of some drugs, whereas kaphas tend to be slow metabolizers, directly in line with traditional Ayurvedic views on their relative digestive power.

Of note, the IGIB study almost didn't happen. As is so often occurs, conventional researchers endeavored to thwart the holistic research. In this case, project reviewers in the institution's Department of Biotechnology turned down the proposal due to their skepticism about Ayurveda. It took more than seven years of persistence by the researchers to finally get the go-ahead, which has validated one of the central tenets of Ayurveda — categorizing individuals on the basis of phenotype.

I am getting stronger and more flexible. As my vitality returns, I am finding myself becoming intrigued by classical hatha yoga techniques. Some of them are discussed in a 14th century practice manual, Svatmarama's *Hatha Yoga Pradipika*, which I recently reread. Many of these practices are rarely taught in yoga classes back home. For example, instead of doing Shoulderstand as I've learned it, with the legs pointing straight up toward the ceiling, I'm doing the more traditional version in which the legs angle up from the torso like a partially opened jackknife. After each exhalation in the upside-down pose, I hold my breath and engage the energetic locks, known as band-has. These techniques are said to direct prana to different areas of the body, or limit its flow in certain directions.

There are three major bandhas. Mula bandha, or root lock, is a subtle lifting up from the center of the pelvic floor. In the solar plexus lock, as you hold the breath out after fully exhaling, you lift the chest as if inhaling — but the glottis stays closed, blocking the inflow of air. The result is a feeling of suction as the abdominal contents are drawn up and in, though in an inverted pose like Shoulderstand, that would be down and in. In chin lock, the chin drops down toward the chest, natural in this pose. With each inhalation, I imagine pranic energy flowing down toward the base of the spine. With each exhalation, I visualize that prana as bright white light, flowing from the root to the third eye.

My sense is that engaging the bandhas facilitates a chaining effect throughout the fascia, and not just in poses. When I engage all three simultaneously, which I do while suspending my breath after each exhalation in my pranayama practice, I can feel a subtle lengthening from the base of my spine to the crown of my head. I see bandhas as being pranic intensifiers, so I'm careful when

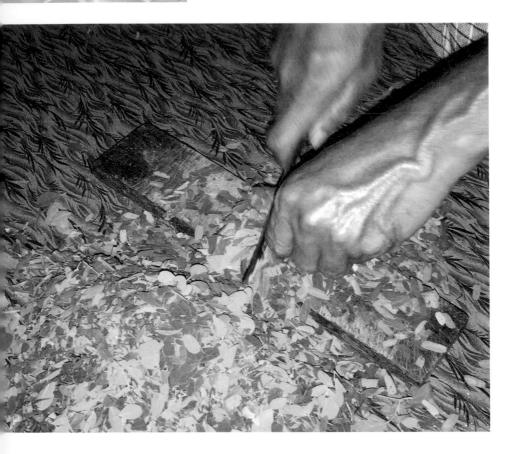

I employ them in pranayama. I only use them when I'm in a retreat setting like this, or when I'm home.

I've always had a twitchy nervous system. If a loud sound comes unexpectedly, I feel a sharp contraction in my solar plexus. It's completely involuntary. Although it was mostly cut off from my awareness at the time, as a kid and younger man, I had tremendous fear — which in a subterranean way colored many of my life decisions. I perseverated about what other people thought of me, and mulled over situations where I worried that I'd not done well in others' eyes. I was always a fragile sleeper, and worrying I might not be able to sleep only made my insomnia worse. These are all characteristic of an excess of vata.

According to Ayurveda, bone problems like mine are also often a manifestation of vata. Focusing on trying to improve my recalcitrant spine, Chandukutty targeted this dosha. I noticed after I returned home that not only did I have an increased range of motion in my spine, I was calmer.

With successive Ayurvedic treatments over the years, and the hundreds of oil massages I've given myself at home between visits to India, my nervous system has continued to change. One way this has manifested is that I now gravitate towards quiet. Back in the States, I used to listen to public radio several hours each day. I'd tape my favorite programs and play them back when I was driving in the car, taking a shower or doing dishes. After my third treatment from Chandukutty, however, I returned to my Bay Area home, looked at the radio in the kitchen, and decided not to turn it on. Even though I'm sure I'm missing some things I would enjoy, I've never gone back.

My experience reflects a crucial Ayurvedic understanding: when you are imbalanced, you tend to make choices that deepen your imbalances; but when you are balanced, your choices help keep you there. My overstimulated brain was always looking for more input, more excitement, more stimulation. As I started to bring my vata down, I chose something that was much better for my jittery nervous system and restless mind: silence.

The slow, smooth breathing that I learned in yoga also helped calm my nervous system. After breathing mindfully for a few years in yoga classes, I noticed that even off the mat, my respiratory rate (RR) hovered at around six breaths per minute.

I don't know for sure what my average breath rate was before yoga. Considering the hyped-up state of my nervous system, I'd guess it was 20 breaths per minute. From a yogic perspective, 20 is not a normal RR — though in modern medicine, 20 is at the high of the normal range. As I would later learn, slow deep breaths are more efficient at delivering oxygen to the lungs than fast, shallow breaths. Faster breathing rates, yoga teaches, also tend to over-stimulate the nervous system and can contribute to problems like insomnia and anxiety, both of which I had.

Scientific research suggests that an RR of six, which became my default — one breath every 10 seconds — has a particularly beneficial effect on the autonomic nervous system (ANS). One study, led by Dr. Luciano Bernardi, of Italy's University of Pavia, examined the effects of chanting either a Sanskrit mantra, Om Mani Padme Hum, or the Latin Ave Maria. Both were found to slow the breath rate to six per minute. This was found to improve two measures of ANS function: heart rate variability and baroreceptor sensitivity.

In a healthy ANS, inhalations will subtly accelerate the heart rate because they stimulate the sympathetic nervous system; exhalations will slow the heart rate back down because they engage the parasympathetic nervous system. That's what causes heart rate variability. Baroreceptor sensitivity relates to how well the blood pressure and heart rate adjust to a quick change in posture, like rising from bed in the morning. Without healthy baroreceptors, on arising, a person might pass out.

Since the ANS directs the functioning of all our internal organs and bodily systems including the cardiovascular, endocrine, and immune systems, improving ANS functioning is potentially valuable in preventing and treating a wide variety of illnesses.

Following the principles of Ayurveda, about ten years ago I taught myself to breathe exclusively through my nose when I exercise — even if it's strenuous exercise. This, I believe, has intensified the calming effects of the slower, deeper breathing I have cultivated. When I first learned this technique, I was guided by a book, *Body, Mind and Sport*, written by the Ayurvedic physician John Douillard. He's taught the technique to world-class athletes, who do it with no loss in their exercise capacity, though the transition typically takes a few weeks. Breathing nasally, they remain calmer and more focused and experience "runner's high" regularly.

One of Ayurveda's most profound insights has to do with chronobiology, the rhythms of nature. When should you get up in the morning? When should you eat the biggest meal of the day? What time should you go to bed? Which foods should you eat in the different seasons? The answers have to do with the rhythms built into nature.

When we align our life with these rhythms, Ayurveda teaches, it's like swimming with the current. When we live our lives out of sync, which modern inventions like electric light, refrigerators, and 24/7 health clubs allow, it's like constantly swimming against the tide. Many of Ayurveda's most valuable lifestyle suggestions have to do with timing: daily, seasonally, and stage of life.

When the sun is at its height in the middle of the day, for example, your agni is at its highest. That's when Ayurveda says that you should eat your largest meal of the day. The worst possible time is when many Americans do it, mid-to-late evening, when kapha dominates. Your agni is at its trough then, and there isn't enough time between finishing your meal and going to bed to digest your meal properly (unless you're retiring at an unhealthily late time).

Going to bed with food still in your stomach, according to Ayurveda, is a formula for the build-up of toxins because the food just sits there, so it doesn't get well-digested. Worse, the work that the body is intended to do at that time — maintenance and house-cleaning — doesn't get done.

Regularity of meal times is also important. Agni, they say, is a historical system. If you eat at noon every day, your body prepares for that. In the half an hour or so before noon, it is slowly turning up the burners of the digestive fire, getting prepared for the meal it expects. If that meal doesn't come, you could develop abdominal symptoms, as I used to experience. If you end up eating hours later, when the agni is not prepared, the meal may not be properly digested, leading to ama.

As I lie on the massage table, Krishna stands at its head, leaning over my torso as he works. I notice a strange odor. Krishna always perspires with the labor, but it's usually clean sweat. Today, though, his sweat smells funny. His breath is also unpleasant, and I've never noticed him have either problem before. This is the smell of ama.

I ask to inspect his tongue. He's got slight cracking on the surface, a sign of increased vata, and a thicker-than-normal whitish film on the surface, a sign of ama. Two days ago, he didn't eat lunch until 3:30 p.m., he says, which is what he suspects first threw him off. Yesterday, lunch was delayed until 4:00 p.m.

No amount of bathing or tooth brushing rids the odor of ama from the body. Usually the person who has it is not aware of it unless someone tells him. Had Krishna checked his tongue this morning, he might have spotted the telltale coating.

———

Amrutha greets me from the doorway: "Good morning uncle!" She's wearing wrap-around fleece earmuffs, in desert-storm camouflage. She sighs and places a steel container on the table; it is the milk that will go into the medicines that Krishna cooks fresh each day for my current treatment, called Navara Kizhi.

She places the back of her hand, surprisingly frosty, on my cheek. "It's cold," she bleats. This makes me curious. The news on my phone announces subzero temperatures and an impending snowstorm back in Burlington. I check the temperature here, and guess it must be what you're used to: it's 71 degrees Fahrenheit.

———

Always aware of the full context of what he's dealing with, and not just my primary diagnosis, Krishna spends extra time massaging my left thigh, right above the knee cap. With the thumb, he irons out any kinks he feels in the tissue that resulted from my quadriceps tendon injury and the subsequent surgery.

In both Ayurveda and TCM, it is believed that scars can block the flow of prana or chi. Treatments to open up these blockages, like massaging oil into the thickened tissue, may be recommended. Scars are examples of adhesions in the fascia, the connective tissue that envelops muscles and organs, and thickens into ligaments and tendons. In her MFR work, Ginny has also spent time trying to open the tissue above my left knee.

As Krishna rubs oil over the surgically-repaired leg, I ask him how it looks to him. Functionally, it feels great.

There is nothing I've tried in the previous months, including hiking and serious booty-shaking dancing, that I couldn't do. Though the muscles have grown stronger since the last time I was in Kerala, we both thought that when I arrived two months ago, there was still a divot. We saw a lateral band, maybe an inch wide across the muscle and about two inches above the kneecap, which hadn't filled in yet. That's where the two ends of the ruptured tendon were stitched back together.

"Normal today," Krishna says, placing a hand on either thigh. "Muscles are same. No depression," meaning the divot is now gone. This speaks to me of the power of the work he is doing with me — not to mention the excellent work the orthopedic surgeon did. It amazes me that an atrophied muscle is getting bigger at a time when I am refraining from exercise, beyond walks to the temple and gentle yoga.

Based on my research, I'd been thinking that I was going to need to do something much more vigorous to build back the last of the atrophied muscle. Had it not been for the limitations on my stamina back in Burlington, I likely would have done much more to build my muscles up.

The express purpose of the treatments we just completed — Navara Kizhi, in which a hot oatmeal-like paste was applied to my body and allowed to cool — was to build back tissue. Earlier treatments we did were designed to remove toxins from the body, setting the stage for healthy new tissue growth. Still, I wasn't expecting the Navara to build the muscle on my leg so quickly, especially in the absence of strong exercise.

Soon, however, I do embark on more active muscle building, partly in response to a suggestion from Swami Madhu. The swami had been with us a few weeks earlier, in order to preside over a fire ceremony, a puja. Krishna arranges one each year, the purpose of which is to bestow auspiciousness on his whole family, and on anyone else who attends the ceremony, as I had done. Afterwards, Krishna suggested that I might want to consult with Swami Madhu about my health concerns, so, as Krishna translated, I asked him about my cancer.

The Swami was very optimistic, feeling that my yoga practice would protect me. But he recommended that I add a practice to my daily routine — staring at the morning sun as it comes over the horizon. Yogis believe this practice brings prana into the body, which can facilitate healing. Since the rays at sunset and sunrise are refracted through much more of the atmosphere than when the sun is higher in the sky, yogis consider it safe for the eyes.

Following his suggestion, I start to do the sun gazing each morning. After a few days, I elaborate on the practice by watching the rising sun while standing in an asana known as Goddess pose. I separate my heels about 18 inches, turn my feet slightly out, and bend my knees enough to allow my buttocks to drop several inches toward the floor. Maintaining this stance, as I inhale, I slowly move into what yogis call "cactus arms," raising my hands from a resting position at my sides to head level with my elbows bent to 90 degrees. As I exhale, I lower the arms back down. After several rounds of that, I stay in the pose with my arms up, knees bent, staring at the orange sun peeking between the fronds of a wall of coconut palms.

This is a challenging pose, but I'm helped by all long holds of deep knee bends I did in my chi gung practice before my cancer was diagnosed. The first time I tried it, I held it for one minute, but I've slowly worked up to more than two minutes. It seems like an excellent way to further strengthen my surgically-repaired leg.

What's difficult about staying in the pose is that the thigh muscles contract powerfully and sometimes painfully. To help with this, I try to keep my breath slow and smooth, and my leg muscles as soft as possible. The calm breathing teaches my nervous system and my mind that they can stay relaxed, even when something unpleasant is unfolding, which is excellent training for life off the yoga mat.

I sit on a small platform, toward the back of the temple, where I pray and do yogic breathing, before meditating on my Durga mantra. When I finish, I cross my hands in front of my chest and try to feel the love of the Mother entering my heart and circulating all throughout me as I exhale. After several breaths, I imagine the loving energy of the Goddess going out to everyone in the temple each time I exhale. On subsequent breaths, I imagine that energy going out farther and farther into the world. This to me is praying.

I've noticed that my prayers these days are seldom for myself, but for various people in my life whom I care about — friends and family, people going through hard times. But I also include some who — in the past, anyway — irritated me. Part of my spiritual work, and part of my cancer therapy as I see it, is to let go of any resentments or harsh judgments that I no longer need.

Where I've had conflict with others, I try to acknowledge my own role in it. Even if I believe my transgressions were small in comparison to theirs, I can feel compassion for them. Yes, someone might have been less than stellar in their conduct, but I know that there are karmic reasons for that, and I can feel good about whatever lessons I learned from our interactions.

When you forgive in yoga, you don't necessarily have to let the other person know. Indeed, I pray and wish well for people whom I hope to never see again. This is about my healing, about releasing emotional leg irons that will allow me to move forward more lightly. And whatever its effects on my health, which at this point remain mostly speculative, I feel confident that my overall well-being is immediately improved by it.

As I sit on the edge of the treatment table waiting for Krishna to complete his preparations for today's treatment, Krishna tells me of a rich man with post-stroke paralysis, on whom he has just completed three days of Dhanya Kizhi. The minimum length of time for Ayurvedic treatment, according to what Chandukutty taught us, is 17 days. But the man refused the longer treatment, Krishna suspects, because he doesn't believe in its effectiveness. Even though Krishna knew that three days would be insufficient, he says he felt obliged to comply with the request because the man had been referred by another patient.

Krishna never mentioned a fee to him. The first day the man gave Krishna 100 rupees for the 75-minute treatment, about US$1.50. Krishna's cost for the medicines alone is several times this amount. Worse, the heat involved is hard on his body and he often gets muscle pains, fatigue, and temporary vision problems (which Ayurveda ties to excess pitta) afterwards. The second day the man paid him 200 rupees, the third day 300 rupees. Krishna only tells me this information in response to my direct questions.

Seeing how he allowed this well-to-do man to take advantage of him, I recognize a pattern I hadn't detected before. "Krishna," I say, "could I please take your pulse?"

He puts down the plastic bottle with the fragrant oil he'd been preparing to massage into my scalp, and hands me his wrist. It's just what I thought: suppressed pitta.

Krishna's constitution has a lot of pitta, but he doesn't let his natural fire shine bright. I call it "dousing your own fire." This sometimes happens, I explain, to children who grow up in a household or culture where a bossy, easily frustrated pitta child, prone to flare-ups of temper, is simply not tolerated. In order to survive, these kids adopt a different strategy. They suppress their fiery nature and take on the role of the good child, the helpful child, the smiley-faced agreeable child. Sometimes people with suppressed pitta haven't allowed themselves to express anger, a natural aspect of pitta, in years.

"When I was a child," Krishna says, "I didn't have no," meaning he couldn't say no even when he knew he should. And that problem has persisted into adulthood. I tell him a story of a student I had at a workshop in Canada with suppressed pitta. This woman had a way of making herself almost invisible. Once I spotted her suppressed pitta and described the phenomenon to her, it was like she flipped a switch. She came in two days later and announced to me and everyone else in earshot: "This morning I told my husband, 'No!' I told my son, 'No!' I told my daughter 'No!'"

Krishna laughs. I think he enjoys hearing about someone who found her no.

Not only does this doormat behavior lead to people taking advantage of you, as the rich man had of Krishna, according to Ayurveda it can also cause disease. When the fire isn't allowed to shine, it gets turned inward and can cause deep-seated inflammatory disease and autoimmune conditions. Suppressed pitta, in my experience, is commonly found in people with Parkinson's disease.

Right now, Krishna has little money. His daughter Aiswarya is an honor student who wants to attend Ayurvedic medical college. It would change the whole course of her life if she were able to do so, but right now Krishna can't afford it. "Krishna," I say, "you just took money from Aiswarya's education and gave it to that rich man. You lost money and you damaged your own body for a patient who didn't deserve it. You need to stop doing this."

Some days later, I sit on the edge of the treatment table. Holding the rag he was going to use to wipe the oil off my body, Krishna mentions that this morning he had felt angry with people in his family and it wasn't like him. He isn't sure he understands what's going on, and he seems concerned.

I ask him to tell me about it and he says he'd felt frustrated about something while talking with Bindu early in the day. Later Amrutha wanted permission to go to a friend's house-warming party and he'd said no. It was close to exams, he told her, and she needed to stay home and study. And then he objected to the tight jeans that Aiswarya had put on for her bike ride to the library to study. "They are unhealthy," he told me. Ayurveda favors baggier clothes, which don't constrict the tissues as much.

"Is your concern about her health or is it the modesty of the jeans that worries you?"

He considers this for a moment. "Both things."

"Before your pitta was suppressed, but now it's much better. You are setting more boundaries."

"Yes."

"Pittas by their nature feel more anger and frustration. They judge people around them who they think are not doing things the right way." With their powers of perception, those with a lot of pitta also tend to have the most sensitive BS detectors.

I get him to describe his interactions with Bindu and the girls. He'd spoken firmly but never raised his voice, never used what he calls "bad language." In other words, he had skillfully used the anger he felt to express what he judged to be correct. He didn't make nice and swallow his feelings as good suppressed pittas do.

Krishna says it is not like him to be forceful with his words. But I am convinced that he is now overcoming a dysfunctional habit pattern that had started early in childhood, out of necessity, but that no longer serves him. He is becoming who is truly is — strong, perceptive, clear thinking and, at the right moments, expressive. And, true to his nature, everything he did came out of love.

From the looks of things, he must not have come down too hard on Aiswarya — she arrives on her bike in the late afternoon, smiling broadly, wearing her jeans.

Early one morning a few days later, I heard Krishna's voice from downstairs. He spoke for a couple of minutes in a much more animated fashion than usual. During my massage I ask him what was going on.

"I was not angry," he says. He had seen Amrutha studying in bed — he pantomimes lying down, holding a book open — "and then I noticed she was sleeping." What I heard was his rousing her from bed to get up and study.

"If we have a chance today, I want to take your pulse again," I tell him. It seems like he is no longer dousing his own fire. "Even though you weren't angry, that was still pitta."

After my lunch, I see him on the porch and tell him that I'd like to check his pulse before he eats his own lunch. When the digestive fire ignites at meal times, pitta increases in the pulse, and I want to feel it beforehand.

Using the first three fingers of my left hand, I take his pulse. I push deeply with the tips of all three fingers until the pulse disappears, then lift them up until bumps appear in each finger. That's the level of the deep pulse that signals prakriti. In Krishna's case, I feel the strong lift in the middle finger pulsation that signals pitta. He's also got quite a bit of kapha in his nature. Then I bring my fingers back toward the surface of the skin until the pulse disappears, and then sink my fingers again until the three pulses reappear. This superficial pulse reflects his current balance. When last I'd checked it, maybe a month ago, there was only a blip under the middle finger. Today it is bounding. With just awareness and the power of intention, Krishna appears to have overcome what was likely a lifelong pattern of pitta suppression.

This morning I do Goddess pose while I stare at the sun, visible only when I stand in just the right spot on the upstairs porch. Through a break in the palm leaves, I can just glimpse a starburst of sun's rays, refracted in all directions like needles. I've been staying longer in the pose, trying to work my way up to five minutes at a time.

I've added silent chanting of the Gayatri mantra to this practice. This prayer comes from the Rig Veda, the oldest of Hindu's ancient scriptures, which may be the oldest extant text in any Indo-European language. It is said to convey healing properties. It honors the light of the sun as the source of life on our planet. This is why it seemed like an appropriate embellishment to my morning sun-gazing ritual.

The legs work hard to maintain the posture for so long — but I can hear the pounding of my heart and it's probably never faster than 100 beats per minute. This is another sign that my conditioning and stamina are improving.

————————

Early one morning in my room, I hear devotional music piped over distant loudspeakers. It is still playing hours later while I eat breakfast. Krishna tells me today is Shivaratri, literally the night of Shiva, an important holiday on the Hindu calendar.

I'd once partaken in an all-night Shivaratri celebration at a yoga ashram in the west. We had chanted till dawn, staying up any way we could, and I found the practice powerful. Since I'm here for Ayurvedic healing, though, I know that missing a night's sleep wouldn't be a good idea, so I'm resigned to not going.

I set out for a walk after breakfast, thinking I'll go to the Vishnu temple I usually visit. But as I look up the hill, through the trees I see a red tile roof of a temple off in a direction where I'd never noticed it before. It looks close, and might be the source of the music. Curious, I decide to take a small road that seems to be heading up toward the sound. Gradually the path narrows. At points, it's just red stone steps cut out of the hill. I see one bicycle, but soon it's clear no vehicles ever come this far. It occurs to me that every brick in every house up here was likely carried by hand.

People are sitting on their porches or passing by, and they smile and nod greetings. The temple music is getting louder to one side but I can't find a way to get over there. I walk further up the hill until the music fades. I turn back until I can catch its strains and decide that the most direct route to it is through a coconut field. This takes

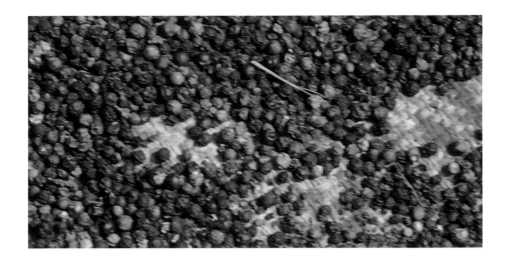

me to what seems like the back entrance of the temple grounds. I take off my flip-flops and, just inside the compound, stop for a moment in front of a collection of snake idols on platforms.

A man in a burnt-orange dhoti approaches. He points me down the hill toward the temple and tells me where to put my chappals, the term locals use for many types of flat footwear. I head toward two small tile-roofed buildings, one of which may be the structure I spotted from the road.

The first building I enter feels full of shakti. I stop in front of an idol and say the Victory Over Death mantra a few times silently. It begins with the word "Tryambakam," Sanskrit for three eyes. That's an allusion to Shiva, who in addition to two normal eyes has a third one, located between his eyebrows. The third eye, yoga teaches, is related to insight and intuition, and can be opened via spiritual practice.

I know the mantra because I recite it 36 times every morning as part of my daily ritual. Chanting it is said to help you overcome fear, including the fear of death. It allows you to let go of attachments, the mantra says, as effortlessly as a cucumber is freed from the vine.

Even great masters, according to yoga texts, still fear their separation from earthly life, and this mantra is one of the most revered and recited. It comes out of the Vedas, and is considered "the heart of the Vedas." The mantra, which is commonly employed as the focus of attention in meditation, is believed to confer healing on those who recite it, silently or aloud, as well as those who hear it chanted.

Mantras gain potency, the tradition says, through repetition. It would not be unusual for a yogi to recite this mantra over a million times. This can take years, though the process is accelerated as the practitioners learn to recite the syllables at breakneck speed. Although I have not come close to repeating the Victory Over Death mantra a million times, it's probably tens of thousands, and I have noticed it feels more powerful and resonant than it initially did.

After my chanting, I go over to the other building, where there is a series of five doors, behind each of which is a stone, bell-jar-shaped Shiva lingam, a phallic representation of God's generative force. The roof is so low that I need to squat to chant here.

As I turn back to the first building, a man tells me that its idol is a female deity — a Devi. I stop and recite my Durga mantra for a good long time. Behind the idol is a poster of a Goddess with weapons in her arms like Durga's. But she has darker skin and a lolling tongue dripping blood, and wears a garland of shrunken skulls around her neck. This is Kali, the Goddess of death, destruction, and sexuality, but also a symbol of motherly love. As I regard the image, I think about Amrutha. That girl's energy is fierce like Kali. The comparison has never occurred to me before, but it feels perfect.

Someone directs me toward the main Shiva temple. As I walk up the hill in that direction, joining a small crowd of others headed the same way, I come upon a smiling woman who speaks to me in English. She asks me if I am here for Ayurveda. I tell her about Krishna.

"I am an Ayurvedic doctor," she says. I inquire about her training. She had attended an Ayurvedic medical college in southern Karnataka, a neighboring state. I ask if she'd had any opportunity to study with a traditional Vaidyar. "My father-in-law is a fifth generation Vaidyar," she says, and she has studied with him. In fact, he is with her today. She points out an elderly man dressed in simple dhoti, wiry with a small belly, and a prodigious mat of white chest hair.

I find myself telling her all about my cancer and treatments, both conventional and holistic, and what has happened to my pulse, in a way I've shared with few others here. "This gives me hope," I say, "modern science and ancient wisdom coming together."

As we arrive, I see a priest, wearing a thin string around his torso, which signals he is a Brahmin. He is carrying brass bowls into the shrine. From what I've observed, usually only the priest enters the inner sanctum. I watch as the elderly Vaidyar follows the priest inside, and ask if others are allowed to go in, too. It was only later that I would learn that this was a private family temple, and that the Ayurvedic doctor was entering with the priest because he was the family's patriarch.

"Go to the fountain and wash your feet," someone says. I raise my feet one by one and run water over them, rubbing them with my hands. A man arrives with a muslin towel, which is to serve as my dhoti. I enter the inner chamber full of dimly-lit ghee lamps, casting their light on an enormous, brass, three-eyed Tryambakam idol. But no one else follows. A small crowd stands outside the door and looks into the shrine.

I sit cross-legged on the bamboo mat they produce for me. The priest begins alternate nostril breathing. I place my fingers to my nose and do the same, opening my eyes a few times to see if I am still on the same step he is. I finish what seems like enough repetitions, and open my eyes to see he has just finished as well. I feel a rush of prana in my head.

The priest balances mini-marshmallow-size camphor chunks on top of several brass ghee lamps. Using a piece of coir string, he lights each chunk and the chamber is illuminated. They burn bright for maybe 30 seconds, and then go out. He slips me a lid of a jar that holds sandalwood powder, into which he has poured a spoonful. I transfer some of the powder from the lid to my right palm and add water, mimicking the priest who is rubbing his hands together to show me I should mix them. Then he points to himself and the Vaidyar and indicates that I should use the thin paste to trace three lines across my forehead, across my heart, and across each of my upper arms, in imitation of the stripes on their own faces, chests, and arms. This is to signal allegiance to Shiva.

The priest's shrill bell echoes. He and the Vaidyar chant. The priest performs an elaborate ceremony made up of hundreds of steps involving picking up flower petals, pouring water into his hands, holding the flowers to his heart, putting them in a brass bowl, and so on. His fingers glide over each other in elaborate gestures, digits overlapping in various configurations, like a classical Indian dancer. He splatters me and the Vaidyar with water, like the priests of my Catholic upbringing.

He begins to chant the Victory over Death mantra rapidly. The Vaidyar is chanting it, too, so I join in for

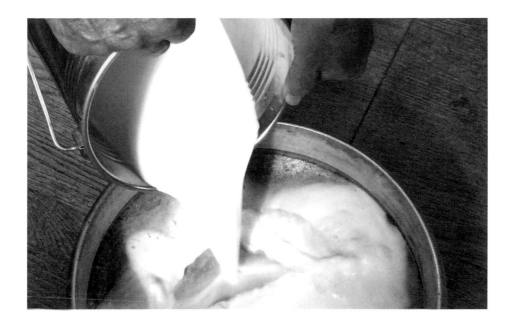

more than a dozen rounds. At such speed and volume, it's an adrenaline rush. I notice the Vaidyar, who had needed to brace himself along the wall as he made his way into the chamber, is looking stronger.

The priest stands up and shuts the door to the small chamber, enclosing the three of us in the oil-lamp light. I have the feeling that I do not belong here, but I try to make the best of it.

The ceremony becomes more elaborate. The priest pours milk over the Shiva lingam. Using his first three fingers, he paints three horizontal lines of sandalwood paste across its base. He places garlands — first of small white flowers, then of orange and yellow marigolds, over the lingam — as well as around the shoulders of the Tryambakam idol.

More bell ringing. As the priest chants, I feel the power of his bhakti, his devotion. Tuning into the rich overtones in his voice, I travel back to my childhood and the Latin Mass. In a way I didn't appreciate then, I now recognize that there was a similar devotion in some of the Catholic chanting I'd heard as a kid.

I find my mind drifting, again feeling like I am someplace I am not supposed to be. Had I acted like a pushy tourist, an entitled foreigner, who'd barged into a sacred space? I know that wasn't my intention, and as I get swept up in the ceremony and the chanting, a strong sense comes over me that this is exactly where I am supposed to be.

Maybe my karma led me to act as I did, and this was the way it was meant to unfold. Why I was permitted inside, I don't know, but it feels like this was karma playing out. That is how I've come to view everything. Every challenge that life has brought me — narcissistic parents, painful relationships, metastatic cancer — is exactly what was meant to be. As is this magical puja on the day of Shivaratri in a temple I found by following my ears.

Once all the milk has been poured on the lingam and all the garlands placed, the priest opens the door. A crowd of women stands out front. Directly in front of the door, an adorable little girl in a velvet dress holds before her a branch of the three-leafed Sriphal plant, evoking the three eyes of Shiva. One leaf, larger and rounder and indented like a ginkgo leaf, sits at the tip of the branch and signifies the third eye. Below it, two smaller leaves stick out to the sides, and signify Shiva's left and right eyes.

Behind the women, in the back and off to one side, stands Krishna. When I was late in returning from my walk, he set out to find me, and in short order he did. When he arrived at the temple, onlookers had told him I was inside. He probably wasn't even surprised I was there, but I was amazed to see him waiting.

As we exit the shrine after the Shiva puja, the old Vaidyar asks if he can take a picture with me. Krishna and another man shoot the photos on their phones. Afterwards, I ask the Vaidyar if he would mind taking my pulse. His daughter-in-law had told me he possesses this skill, though she said she does not. By my reckoning, my pulse has been normal for the last couple of months. But he's likely been assessing the pulse since before I was born. I am fascinated to hear what he thinks.

Standing in front of the shrine, near the statue of Nandi, Shiva's devoted bull, he places three fingers along my right wrist artery. He spends more than a minute, at times slightly adjusting the pressure of his fingers.

"There is no disease," he says. "Healthy pulse."

The Vaidyar's assessment reassures me. So did some news I'd received right before Christmas. Even since last summer, I'd been concerned about the Canadian study, which suggested a much worse than expected prognosis for HPV-related oral cancer. Knowing this, Dr. Clark sent me a study that had just been released. Based on the outcomes of hundreds of patients with HPV-related oral cancers treated at New York's Memorial Sloan Kettering Cancer Center (MSKCC), the study was much more encouraging. At five years, survival rates were just over 85 percent. The 10-year survival rate topped 75 percent — by contrast the Canadian study showed only 18 percent.

MSKCC got better results, it appeared, partly because they used intensity-modulated radiotherapy. IMRT's improved equipment allows the radiation to more precisely target the cancerous tissues, while to some degree sparing normal tissues. In the past, treatments sometimes failed because the beam missed its mark; IMRT reduces such failures almost to zero. I feel confident that the treatment

I received was comparable in quality to MSKCC's. It's true that the study included people with tumors at all stages, I-IV, and that my own risk of recurrence with a IVa tumor is likely higher than the study's average, but this was still very encouraging news. And, of course, I hope that everything I did — including the fasting during treatment — improved my odds.

Dr. Clark concluded his note by wishing me happy holidays. I couldn't have asked for anything better for Christmas.

Even Krishna's family has a temple. Years ago, a relative agreed to allow one to be built on a corner of his personal property, for the use of the entire extended family. The temple complex, which I saw several years ago, is modest and made up of several improbably small buildings. They had fallen into disrepair, though, and it was Krishna who led the campaign to renovate them.

The work is almost done, and in preparation for the ceremony that will follow, Krishna is about to begin a period of tapas, Sanskrit for penance, austerity, discipline. Fish is a staple of the diet in Kerala, but for the next 41 days, he'll eat none. He'll also chant more mantras than usual.

He tells me that he plans to cut all his hair off as well. I ask if he would like to borrow the electric clippers I brought with me. We find a place in the upstairs hall to plug them in. The cord is just long enough to reach out to the brightness of the balcony.

"Would you like me to cut it for you?" I ask. He says yes. We spread an old newspaper on the floor, and I set to work, buzzing away at the sides. His thick, wavy, graying-to-white hair falls in chunks. For fun, I leave the top of his head untouched. This conservative 50-something

Hindu now sports the very same look I've seen on a couple of the cooler teenage boys around town. *I've got to get a picture of this.* I dash to my room and grab my phone.

"Hold on," I say, "I want to show these to the girls." It's amazing. The wrong hair style looks so right on him. This could go on a magazine cover. He is striking.

Downstairs, I show Aiswarya the image. Her mouth drops open and she lets out a laugh that sounds more like a cough. Next is Amrutha, who cries out, eyes widening with glee. Their father, with that cool haircut, does not fit into the world they thought they knew.

I go back upstairs, the girls following eagerly. Amrutha and Aiswarya are beside themselves as they first lay eyes on Krishna. They watch as I remove the rest of his hair. By now, the boys have joined us.

"Appu wants," Aiswarya says, indicating her cousin. It seems he's sold on the cut that looked so good on Krishna. *What the heck.* I agree. Appu, who is now 11, takes his place on the newspaper.

Appu's hair, though, is not the luxuriant kapha hair that Krishna has. It's straighter and finer, more pitta-like, and much less forgiving if cut poorly. I begin to worry that I might be giving him a bad haircut. I keep my doubts to myself and proceed. The girls chime in with occasional advice. If not for them, one side of Appu's hair might now be longer than the other.

Finally, the cutting is done. Appu is happy he's been treated to the kind of haircut his parents would never spring for. The girls are happy to have been part of the experience. And I'm just happy it's over.

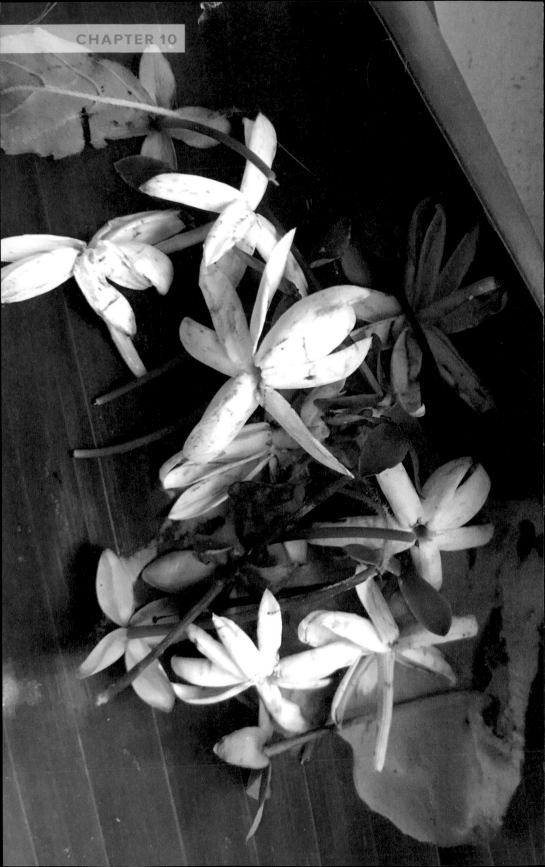

CHAPTER 10

"When the breath is unsteady, the mind wanders. When the breath quiets, the mind is calm, and the yogi may live a long life."

— Svatmarama

HOLDING MY BREATH

It is the second day of the annual festival at the Mahasudarshana temple. A band of musicians stands out front under a canopy, generating an insistent, almost frenzied beat. About a dozen drummers in two lines play long drums, hanging from their left shoulders. They wield sticks in both hands, going at it in unison, elbows at their sides, cranking their forearms up and down as if playing a drum roll. In their midst an old man clacks a pair of hand-held pewter-colored cymbals in front of his chest on each beat.

Facing them is the horn section. Half a dozen men play horns with brass-colored stems looping up and back toward them in perfect half-circles. They move in synchrony like The Pips, performing with attitude for the drummers. They bend forward and snap back up, elbows bent, shoulders twisting to the side as they descend, and twisting back as they come up.

I watch for a couple of minutes, less bothered by the volume than yesterday, before I head into the temple where the sound is muffled. Despite the crowd out front, there are few people inside. I sit in my customary place on the platform in the back and begin my mantra meditation.

Walking home, I hear a noise pounding as insistently as the drums I'd just heard. Bhummm, bhummm, bhummm. I realize it's the sound of my feet, one after the other, striking the ground in front of me. I must have been hearing this sound throughout my life, but I never noticed it before — precisely, I presume, because it was always there. When I straighten my knees fully as I step, the sound is sharper. When I keep a slight bend in the knees, it's softer and more watery. Walking this way feels better. This is the same realization I've come to in my yoga practice: keeping a slight bend in the knees makes all the poses feel better.

It occurs to me that this sound — always there but unnoticed — is analogous to the rhythm that greeted us as we first developed our ability to hear in the womb. Buh BHUMM, buh BHUMM, buh BHUMM — the double-beat rhythm of mother's heart, resonating through the amniotic fluid, and in every cell of the unborn child. I suspect I suffered from the absence of that soothing rhythm as I lay in the incubator. Now, when it's quiet and I sit in meditation, I hear the same drumbeat coming from my own heart.

Before dawn, Krishna and I ride to the oceanfront in Calicut for a puja to honor the one-year anniversary of Chandukutty's death. We take an auto-car, the latest automotive trend here. It's got an auto-rickshaw's two-stroke motor, but has four wheels instead of three. Rather than being open on the sides, it's enclosed by a thin metal exterior with two doors on one side and one on the other.

We meet the priest on the beach. Holding a broad LED light that penetrates the darkness, he guides us to a spot near where waves lick the shore. We change into the dhotis we brought with us, not the usual dress ones that extend to our ankles, but instead pieces of paper-thin muslin that wrap around our waists and reach almost to our knees. Behind us, in a pit deep enough to protect the flame from the wind, a ghee lamp provides soft illumination.

The priest begins the ritual with a long chant that I recognize, an invocation of Ganesha. Using a traditional gesture, we straighten the fingers of our right hands, and pick up rice, sesame seeds, and flower tops. The priest guides us through a series of complicated steps that I find hard to follow. I get through it with cues from Krishna and the priest. We hold the offerings between our hands in prayer position as the priest intones a mantra. His chanting reminds me of the enthusiastic, endearing, and slightly out-of-tune voice in which Chandukutty used to sing devotional songs for company, unbidden.

The priest tells us to visualize Chandukutty, and then our own ancestors, as we pray. Standing, each of us holds a piece of palm leaf heaped with offerings of flowers, ghee, herbs, sandalwood paste and black sesame seeds. We turn clockwise three times, then drop the leaves over our heads behind us onto the sand. These offerings are meant for the birds.

Krishna and I pick up two more banana leaves, sagging with offerings, and carry them over to the water. Krishna steps into the warm waves and I follow. Ship lights are visible on the black horizon. We turn to face the shore and lift the leaves over our heads with both hands and drop them behind us. The undertow carries them out to sea.

Riding home in the auto-car, I am struck by how sad Chandukutty Vaidyar's life always seemed to me. He'd

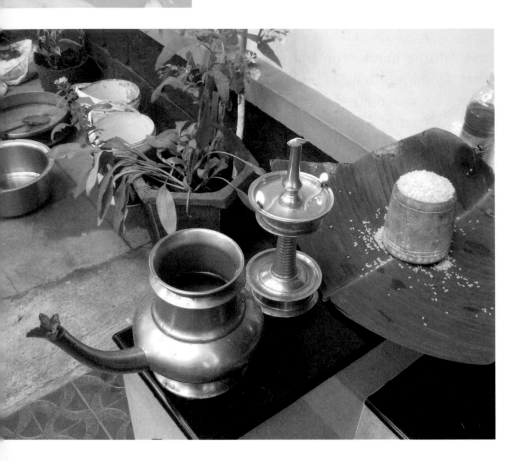

been estranged from most of his children for years, and they'd only reconciled late in his life. He lived alone, in a dark house, with stacks of dusty papers and closets full of empty medicine bottles. He had stacks of fancy dhotis — gifts from patients — more than anyone could ever wear. He'd died wealthy, yet Krishna once told me that Chandukutty rarely spent any of his money.

As sad as I was to see Chandukutty die without having passed most of his knowledge on, it occurs to me that must have been much harder for him to bear. He may have also been depressed to see the state of Ayurveda in India. Even though its popularity has been growing, in his eyes most of it was inauthentic. He believed most of the oils and herbal medicines sold in stores were of low quality. Adding insult, the Indian government had required that Chandukutty keep a licensed Ayurvedic doctor — which he was not — on staff, in order for him to practice his art legally. That meant he had to hire a graduate of Ayurvedic medical college — who couldn't have known a tenth of what he knew — to oversee his work. I met two of these doctors over the years. Soon after each was hired, they had prostrated themselves before Chandukutty and humbly asked to become his student.

"How do you think Vaidyar would feel about the ceremony," I ask.

"I think he is happy," Krishna says. I hope he is right.

———————————

After returning from the puja, Krishna recounts his early days with Chandukutty. "It was just the two of us every evening in Kochi," he says. For many months, Vaidyar didn't pay him, but because Krishna viewed him as his guru, he accepted that. Krishna treated eight or ten patients a day, working late into the evenings, then cooked for Chandukutty and himself.

Even once Chandukutty gave him a monthly salary, it was never enough to meet expenses. His brother Manoj supported the family while Krishna was gone, doing what he could, but some days the kids ate little more than rice. There was no money for curry or fish. Each child got two dates and two cashews per day, the latter ritually doled out by their paternal grandfather, who also took only two of each. Meanwhile, Chandukutty's business was booming and he was becoming by local standards a wealthy man. This went on for 14 years, during which time Krishna was allowed to return home to his family for only one or two days per month. After eight years, Chandukutty opened an additional clinic near Calicut, where he and Krishna started spending a couple of days per week — which at least allowed Krishna to sleep at home those nights.

What made Krishna stay through all of this? Part of it was the patients. Most were chronically ill and had tried allopathic doctors, or visited Ayurvedic hospitals without finding relief. Yet often within a few days, Krishna reports, they were noticeably better — and deeply grateful. He had the sense that he was supposed to be there.

He probably also stayed because of what he was learning, not that Chandukutty cared about that — he never taught Krishna any more than he needed to. These so-called "hereditary Vaidyars" hold their family secrets tightly, and offer only tidbits to students. But whenever Vaidyar — as Krishna always refers to his teacher — had a patient with some complex illness or bodily finding that Krishna didn't know how to respond to, Chandukutty would show him what to do. With his hands he'd demonstrate exactly how to modify the massage techniques, or tell Krishna how to adjust the preparation methods for the medicines.

Over their years together, Krishna learned a lot, including how to give all the major treatments, as well as the traditional methods to prepare the oils and herbal remedies. Vaidyar was a master at perceiving what was going on with his patients, and Krishna picked up some of that as well. And although Chandukutty never encouraged it, Krishna read books on Ayurveda to better understand what he was doing.

Even Chandukutty's brother, a schoolmaster who also knows Ayurveda, recommended that Krishna quit. But I suspect a comment Krishna made in another context might best explain why he stayed loyal: "My name is not

Krishna. It is Krishna Dasan." He meant that he is not God, but God's servant. His dharma, or life purpose, as he sees it, is to serve. A life of service is what's known as Karma yoga, the path of action. You do your dharma, with no expectation of receiving anything in return.

––––––––––––––

Krishna stands at the head of the massage table and ties a mud pot to a rope, looped through a hook mounted on the ceiling. A braided cotton wick sticks out through a hole in the bottom of the pot. Krishna leans a pan containing medicated buttermilk against the edge of the vessel and pours in the beige liquid. We are beginning the next stage of my treatment, Dhara — the drizzling of cool buttermilk over the third eye. This has been my favorite Ayurvedic treatment ever since my first trip to Kerala.

"You know," Krishna says, "every Shiva temple has a Jala Dhara," Sanskrit for a flowing stream or waterfall.

"For the visitors or for the idol?"

"For the idol." Shiva spends so much time in meditation that his brain can overheat, Krishna explains. The stream of water cools his pitta and helps him stay balanced.

Even the gods, it would seem, need Ayurveda.

Having completed his preparations, Krishna adjusts the wick and sends the buttermilk careening down toward the middle of my forehead, at first in spurts, then a smooth flow. As the streaming liquid first lands, I shudder from the cold, experiencing a jolt, like the beginning of an ice cream headache. It feels as if the buttermilk must have been refrigerated, but I know that's not possible in this house. Even though I don't enjoy the liquid's temperature, I imagine it as cooling excess pitta in my brain as well as my body, which yesterday had a pitta elevation due to a brief intestinal infection.

Allowing the pot to gently swing from the rope so that the buttermilk flows in a side-to-side stream above my brow, Krishna begins with his other hand to massage my forehead and scalp. This is the most delicious part of every Dhara treatment, instantly taking me into a relaxed state. Already the buttermilk is feeling warmer.

During Dhara, I ask Krishna to try an experiment. Would he please massage the line from the third eye between the eyebrows up the skull's midline toward the anterior fontanelle? That's the residual of the soft spot babies have above their foreheads. It feels good when he does it, but not amazing. I ask him to push harder, but discover that with Dhara, and the deep nervous system relaxation it induces, slow and tickle-light feels best.

As he moves back down toward the third eye, the sensation heightens. I ask him to massage me a bit lower, right between the eyebrows. To do so, he needs to move the thick cotton rope that is wrapped from ear to ear across my forehead, which keeps the buttermilk from leaking into my eyes. As he moves his thumb in clockwise direction (from his perspective), I exhale deeply. Mmmmmmm.

"Krishna, you have to include this every time you do Dhara," I say. "That's a marma point, right?

"It's the first marma," he says, meaning the most important. "Everything comes in the body through this point."

"Could you try to massage it in the other direction?" I say, anti-clockwise, as they call it here. After three or four strokes I tell him it's not right and to please go back to clockwise.

"We are always massaging only in this direction," he says.

"We have our ideas, and sometimes they are good ones," I say, "but the body knows more than we do."

"When I am massaging the body, it tells me where it needs the attention."

I ask him to try the area around the anterior fontanelle. Again, he moves in a small clockwise circle. I can feel my whole body sinking into the wood table. Goose bumps rise from head to toe. I exhale deeply again and again. "Is that also a marma point?"

"Yes."

"Could you try the posterior fontanelle?"

"Sure." He massages in the same way toward the back of the scalp but I don't feel anything special. He moves up toward the crown of the head, which feels nice but nothing like the first two marma points he'd massaged. I reach my hand back to feel for the posterior fontanelle, a slight depression where the skull bones knitted together early in life.

I finger the soft spot toward the back of the head, and realize his aim had been off. "Here," I say, holding the tip of my finger on it so he can see exactly where it is. Krishna begins to trace clockwise circles around this point and a wave of relaxation hits. Goose bumps again.

"I think we just discovered something that the ancients had to have known about. Didn't Chandukutty ever talk about this?"

"People here are only talking about how high the pot should be or how fast the buttermilk flows."

At the two other Ayurvedic centers in Kerala I'd been to, they had also massaged the scalp during Dhara, but not as well or to the extent that Krishna does. Krishna has honed his perceptive abilities via the thousands of Ayurvedic treatments he's given, and his years of practicing Kerala's indigenous martial art Kalari as a child. I, in turn, have practiced tens of thousands of hours of yoga, and had hundreds of sessions of various styles of bodywork, as well as many months of Ayurvedic treatments. Together, Krishna and I were able to take something passed on to us from our teacher, Chandukutty Vaidyar, and take it deeper.

Chandukutty may well have been aware of what we've discovered, but if so, he never taught it to Krishna. This is not some technique that Krishna and I invented. Rather, it is something built into our bodies and nervous systems that we got quiet and curious enough to find.

This is a small example of exactly how yogis have figured out all the amazing things they have been discovering for millennia. The ancient sages of Ayurveda, just like the rishis of yoga, had heightened their powers of perception through years of meditation and other practices — and it was from that vantage point that they were able to tune into their bodies with such sensitivity. And that's also how they tuned into what was happening in their patient's bodies.

Krishna's and my discovery of those three sweet spots on the skull has transformed the oil massages he is giving me, as well as the ones I give myself on the days he's not available. The relaxation is deeper, similar to what I experience with Dhara treatments. Sometimes it only takes seconds of rubbing those spots for the relaxation to wash over me. It's more profound when Krishna does it to me, but still amazing when I do it myself.

I'm used to relaxing deeply. It's a state that you have to work up to. Shavasana, I find, doesn't typically get really good till about 10–15 minutes in. Most people never stay long enough in the pose to discover that. But with this marma massage, I sink deep in seconds. I'm sure there's a biologic correlate to what I'm feeling, maybe a natural opiate being released, and I would love to know what it is. But in the meantime, my lived experience is all the proof I need.

─────────────

Lately the focus in my pranayama practice has been on expanding my breath capacity — that is, learning to breathe ever more slowly — and to suspend the breath for longer periods of time. Due to the chemoradiation I became anemic, and last I heard my blood count, and therefore my oxygen carrying capacity, was still down 15-20 percent from what it had been. It improved only slightly between my three-month and six-month post-treatment checkups. This was a big part of why I backed off on my breath retentions in pranayama during my cancer treatment and afterwards. But now I find that I'm able to resume longer breath holding.

Alternate nostril breathing has been the primary vehicle I've used over the years to gradually build my ability to hold the breath. Known as Nadi Shodhana, which means, "cleansing the energetic pathways," it's the practice that Hillary Clinton described and Dr. Hamblin ridiculed. In the version I'm doing every day, I inhale, hold my breath, exhale, and hold again — each for the same number of seconds. This pattern is called Square Breathing. I keep count with my Durga mantra, which takes about four seconds to recite silently. I chant two Durga mantras in a row for each part of the four-part sequence, so each breath takes just over 30 seconds. Slow acclimation over years of practice allows me to do this without any strain, even in the face of significant anemia.

This is a profoundly calming and grounding practice, as long as you have slowly built up your breath capacity and can do it comfortably. There should never be any gasping or any breath hunger. Although it may not look like much, this pranayama is strong and if you haven't prepared for it, it can mess up your nervous system and even lead to a mental breakdown.

Yoga teaches that alternate nostril breathing enables you to breathe equally through both nostrils, which facilitates attaining a meditative state. Thus, Nadi Shodhana is considered to be the perfect preparation for meditation, allowing you to go more quickly into a quiet, less-distracted state of mind. I'm finding it ever more effective and, even after 18 years, I sense the potential to go deeper.

―――――――――――

I watch a video on my laptop of the yoga guru Krishnamacharya, filmed in 1938, when he was 50. In recent years, it has been his later-life students — including his son, TKV Desikachar, and AG Mohan — who have been most influential in my practice, especially the breath retention work I've been doing. Krishnamacharya was also BKS Iyengar's guru. In the grainy black-and-white film, his body looks both taut and lithe. There are gray hairs on his temples and in his scruffy beard, but his physique could be that of a man of 20. He flows from one challenging yoga pose to another, always appearing at ease.

Although I've seen the film before, something strikes me as I watch it this time that I don't remember. Krishnamacharya is sticking his tongue down and way out every time he activates the three bandhas, the energetic locks. Holding his breath out after an exhalation, he lifts up his abdomen and puffs out his chest in a mock inhalation, while lowering his chin toward his chest, thrusting his tongue down. I've done this practice thousands of times, but never with my tongue out.

I decide to try it. I stand up and, bending my knees

deeply, place each palm on its respective thigh. After emptying my lungs, I expand my chest as if I were inhaling, without bringing any air in, then stick out my tongue while lowering my head. I feel a connection between the suction in my abdomen, and the soles of my feet. During long holds of the breath with empty lungs, I move my tongue side-to-side and notice how I can use its movement to open distant areas of the body.

As I let go of the locks and stand up, sadness envelops me. I take the emotion in, focusing on where it lives in my body. Behind my eyes, I feel moisture, as if a precursor of tears.

I try Downward-Facing Dog pose, my body in a V-shape, with my buttocks in the air and my hands and feet on the floor. Lately I've been doing this pose with a deep knee bend, as I find it facilitates more freedom in my spine. Once again, I engage the bandhas and stick my tongue out as far as it will go, holding my breath out. As I inhale and come out of the pose, another wave of sadness rolls over me.

This emotion is powerful, yet, as has happened several times in the last year, there is no story attached. I don't feel sad about anything in particular. It is just a powerful bodily sensation that I identify as sadness. Yoga teaches that emotions can live in bodily tissues; in this case it would seem in my tongue.

I do a wide variety of poses and discover that sticking the tongue out and down, as Krishnamacharya had done, deepens the bandhas and facilitates forward bending. I go deeper into several of these asana than I ever have in my life. And after each pose, another wave of sadness arrives. I pause and watch that for a couple of minutes then do another pose.

Although the dominant emotion is sadness, at times

it is tinged with anger. Sometimes when I close my eyes and look inside, I see blackness, which I've experienced other times when difficult emotions arise in my practice. My sense is that whatever this is, it is old and deep. Since there's no story attached, I'm wondering if this could be related to preverbal trauma, perhaps what happened to me in childbirth and its aftermath.

I sit on my heels, with my toes turned under like a sprinter's, and the soles of my feet facing the wall behind me. This is a strong stretch for the feet. When I first did it in yoga classes, it hurt, but years later it's become comfortable. From there, I pitch my torso slightly forward, and my hands press into the thighs for Lion's pose. This is a crazy-looking traditional hatha yoga pose that I've been doing recently. You cross your eyes toward the midline, thrust your tongue out, and roar like the king of the jungle. Mine sounds more like a growl.

Sticking my tongue out, I suspend my breath and engage the bandhas. That tongue action triggers something like a lightning bolt. I feel the connection via the myofascia from my tongue to my diaphragm to the base of my pelvic floor, and all the way down to the big toe side of each foot. I breathe deeply, near tears.

When I settle into Corpse pose, lying back on the floor, all traces of the sadness are gone. I sink in.

When I stand up, my feet feel broad and heavy on the floor. I wonder for a second whether I might have lost my normally strong arches, as so much of my foot seems to be in contact with the ground. I reach down and reassure myself that my arches are just fine.

The next day I experience just a little sadness when I attempt some of the same poses with my tongue extended. In the days that follow, I use my tongue to deepen the bandhas, but the emotions never return.

Dr. Kuantai — the Vermont ear, nose and throat doctor — recommended that I follow up with her in three months. I'll be gone longer than that, so I decide to get some blood tests, including thyroid function tests (TFTs), and a complete blood count. I'm especially interested in the TFTs, hoping that the abnormal results from Burlington have improved and that the gland might be spared. Last fall, after I'd completed my treatment, my TFTs were abnormal. What I'd read led me to fear that I was headed for full-blown hypothyroidism.

Once again, Krishna and I take an auto-car taxi, driven by his neighbor. We arrive at the testing center, which Krishna researched on my behalf. He says it's the best one in Calicut. In the lobby, a man directs me to join a short line. I hand my handwritten list of tests through the glass to a clerk who scrolls through his computer, finding each test I've requested. Most of the people in the lines beside me are clutching handwritten prescriptions from their doctors indicating which tests they need. But anybody here can have any test they can pay for. No one asks for an ID.

The clerk asks my name. After I pronounce it, he asks me to write it in on the paper I've given him. I print Dr. Timothy. Nobody here uses last names, and I figure the Dr. part won't hurt. It comes to 2,300 rupees, about $35. The same tests back home cost me more than ten times that amount.

Inside, the blood drawing room is clean and modern. A technician expertly sticks my arm with a disposable needle and withdraws three tubes of blood. I'll be able to look up the results on their website in four hours. She leaves me with a cocoa brown polka dot bandage over my pink elbow crease. This strikes me as only fair after so many brown brothers and sisters have endured lifetimes of Band-Aids the shade of the "skin color" crayon in my childhood box of 64.

The kids are gathered in the hall outside the kitchen when we get back. Aiswarya approaches me, holding the black kitten by the back of the neck. "Look uncle," she says. "It's Litu Bieber!"

Whenever she says this name in her sweet accent, I hear, "Little Bieber," and it makes me smile.

Appu pets Litu Bieber as Aiswarya holds it. I join in, running a finger over its small head. I hold my finger in front of its dry nose so it can smell me, which it does with careful consideration.

"Has anyone figured out if it is a boy or girl?" I ask. Amrutha doesn't understand. "Do you know if it is male or female?"

"I DOONE know," she says.

I lift the kitten's hind leg, revealing small nipples on her lower belly. "It's a girl," I say.

"Uncle," Aiswarya says, "It's making a sound. What is it?"

I put my ear close to the kitten. "She's purring. P, U, R, R," I spell, and I explain what it means when a cat does that.

About to lie down for Shavasana one morning, after my usual breath capacity-building asana practice, I think of Pop. We were at the lake house. I was maybe ten. He'd been writing about B.F. Skinner, the chief propagator of behaviorism, who believed we all come into the world with a clean slate. All our actions, behaviorists maintain, are the result of some behaviors being reinforced and others not.

When we'd driven to Vermont that summer, we'd brought along our cat, who had set never foot outside the house. After we arrived, we let him out of the car. Free to roam the wooded area surrounding the lake house, he returned within minutes with a bird in his mouth. Skinner's theory, Pop insisted, couldn't explain that.

As I settle into the pose, I find myself thinking about Pop's terrible pride. He was brilliant and way ahead of his time in understanding many things, but he constantly felt the need to demonstrate how smart he was.

A feeling of shame washes over me. I sense fullness behind my eyes, which extends down the jaw line. But this feels like Pop's emotion, not mine. The shame morphs into sadness. My eyes constrict and well up. My tongue pushes to the roof of my mouth. That sadness becomes tinged with fear. There is tightening deep in my lower abdomen.

As the emotion starts to wane, I find myself silently chanting my Durga mantra. As I inhale, I imagine the love of the Mother coming into my heart. As I exhale, I send that love, flowing out to Pop.

I check my blood tests online. My blood count has returned to a shade below 40 — essentially normal — up from 35 four months ago. That number hadn't budged much from three months to six months after chemoradiation. Could my efforts to build breath capacity have played a role in this improvement? Low oxygen levels spur the production of red blood cells. That's why people living at altitude have higher blood counts.

My lymphocyte count, a type of white blood cell related to immune function, remains low close to a year out from treatment. I'm told that may persist. Clinically, though, my immune function continues to be good. Several members of Krishna's family have been sick while I've been here and I've managed to not get any of it. And even when I got food poisoning — from eating a single grape I mistakenly believed had been washed — I was fine the next day.

Best of all, my thyroid function has returned to normal. If I've somehow managed to escape chemoradiation with my thyroid intact, that would be amazing.

———————————

While looking for a photo on my laptop today, I open a file that turns out to be a selfie of my ex. Such unexpected reminders happen often; our lives were so intertwined.

We were best friends and lovers, ate almost all our meals together (usually she cooked and I cleaned up the mess, which when she got inspired could be prodigious). We shared a passion for yoga, practiced together in our home studio, traveled and taught yoga therapy seminars together, and ran a yoga therapy center (although that was her baby more than mine).

While I haven't always appreciated these random visitations since our breakup, today's is not unwelcome. As I contemplate her inviting smile and stare into her eyes, I silently say to her, *What a beautiful mess we made.*

Since we split, I have done a lot of psychological work and owned my role in that mess. Without going into my traditional pattern of moving past the pain too quickly, I made space for the emotions I needed to feel — sadness, anger, shame at the failure of the relationship — so as to let them go and find peace.

While the marriage cost me some heartache and some money, I have no regrets. I learned so much from the relationship and its aftermath. After years of being what is known in India as a "chronic bachelor," I'd finally gotten married. I doubt that would have happened were it not for all the work I'd done to open my heart. Though I was blind-sided by the breakup, within a few months, I began to see a few things I had missed. I came to understand that she'd done me a big favor.

———

I have been trying to sort out whether after successfully bringing my vata back to normal, I am going too far the other way — over the line into kapha excess. My body feels heavy. I lie in bed as if encased in wax, as my alarm plays the Victory Over Death mantra, chanted by Shubhra, on repeat.

But the signs point to balance. My pulse is smooth and watery, with no abnormal spikes anywhere, just three strong pulses in the vata, pitta, and kapha fingers.

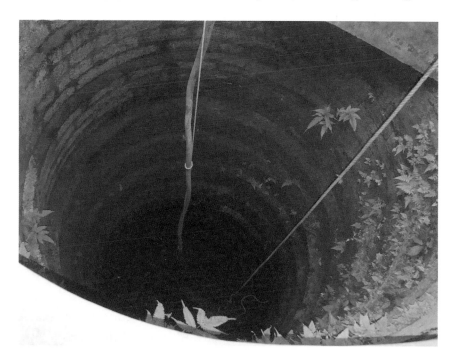

I examine my tongue in the mirror every morning — it is clean and smooth, with no abnormal coating. Like many people with a lot of kapha in their constitution, I may not feel like exercising but once I begin, I have good endurance. I clocked my Goddess pose this morning at five minutes. Lately that five-minute hold hasn't felt that demanding.

Then it dawns on me. This is what being grounded feels like. It's only strange because it is foreign to my experience. Even though it's taking me longer than usual to get out of bed, I kind of like it. I could get used to living like this, moving more slowly but feeling more earthy and stable.

———————————

Aiswarya arrives home from her exam review course in Calicut while I am sitting on the front porch. She has been reminding me over the last several days that she would like to do a session of yoga therapy with me.

"Aren't you too busy?" I ask.

"I'll make the time," she says.

Aiswarya is about to eat dinner, so I suggest we start with taking her pulse now, before eating changes it. Her prakriti, her constitution, is pitta vata, with strong beats felt with my index and middle fingers on the deep pulse. Although the entire family has an abundance of pitta, she's got the most vata, which is reflected in her thin frame and wavy, sometimes frizzy, hair.

I am not surprised by her superficial pulse, which indicates her current state of balance. Her vata is sky-high, consistent with the headaches she's been suffering and her recurring anxiety, most recently about her test performance. But, as I'd suspected, pitta is nowhere to be found. Like her father, Aiswarya can be too nice, too accommodating. She is another suppressed pitta.

As we talk, I am covertly watching her breathing. When I do yoga therapy assessments, my plan is to observe some things before the student figures out what I'm looking at — because otherwise they might change what they do. Something seems to be off with her breath, but I haven't figured it out yet. Her baggy salwar kameez top doesn't help.

"In our course, there was a chapter on breathing," she says. "When the diaphragm moves down, the belly pushes out. But I noticed I was doing the reverse." That's it. She's a paradoxical breather. I've never had a student who'd noticed it before I did.

"I want to show you a video," I say. "I'll be right back." I unplug my laptop in my room and bring it down to the porch.

I click the first video. The woman, in profile, draws her abdomen in toward her spine on each inhalation and pushes it back out on the exhalation. Then we watch a video of her breathing in the way I taught her. Her abdominal muscles contract on the out breath to squeeze more air out, and her belly pooches out as she breathes in. Aiswarya can see the difference between the two.

"Now watch again. This time I want you to look at her face as she breathes." In the first clip, at the end of each inhalation, the woman's eyes bulge and she lifts her eyebrows as if she were frightened. It looks like each inhalation brings a spritz of adrenaline. As she exhales, her smile looks more like a grimace. She's probably breathing that way due to stress — and it's a self-reinforcing feedback loop — as the paradoxical breathing jacks up her fight or flight response.

In the second video, her eyes bulge with the first breath. As she gets into a rhythm with belly breathing, though, her eyelids start to get heavy and flutter down like those of a toddler insisting that she doesn't need a nap. "Can you see the difference in what those two breathing styles are doing to her nervous system?" Aiswarya nods. "That's what you're doing. Can you see why you might have anxiety?"

Yes, she says.

"This is good news," I say, "even though it might not seem like it. You've got suppressed pitta and paradoxical breathing, two of the fastest conditions to respond to yoga therapy." Both imbalances lead to increased vata, I explain, which fuels pain and a distracted, worried mind.

Then I play my trump card. "I think fixing your breathing could help you remember what you're studying better. You'll also be more relaxed when you take your exam."

———

To try to understand paradoxical breathing better, I study the videos I'd shown Aiswarya. The more times I watch them, the more I learn.

There are two main movements of the ribs in healthy chest breathing. The upper ribs lift up as the breath comes in, and the lower ones move back and out to the sides. In the video, when the woman breathes paradoxically, she only does the former, and in a jerky fashion no less.

I try it myself, contracting my abdomen on each in-breath, and letting it go on the exhalation. It feels terrible. I put my palms on the sides of my lower ribs. Just as I'd observed in the video, there is no movement on the inhalation. After only a minute of breathing this way, I become agitated. No wonder Aiswarya's been anxious and in pain. She's probably been doing this for years.

In four years of medical school and three years of residency training, I never heard anyone talk about paradoxical breathing. Even the idea that dysfunctional breathing could in any way influence symptoms or disease processes was never discussed. Yoga teaches that there are various breathing dysfunctions that can cause problems. And from what I've seen in my yoga therapy work, when you can re-pattern such a person's breath, there can be major improvements in their health and well-being — sometimes rapid.

A few days later, I finally do a yoga therapy session with Aiswarya, while Krishna observes. We work in the upstairs hall, which has the most space, though it's darker than optimal. I start by evaluating her structure, walking around her as she stands to assess her from different angles.

Krishna watches from his seat on the floor but I suggest he get up and come behind Aiswarya to see what I am seeing. Not wanting her to be influenced, I silently point to her heels, tracing a line of dysfunction up past her ankles with my finger. I also alert Krishna to the protrusion of her right shoulder blade and a subtle rotation of her upper torso. He nods, letting me know he sees what I'm indicating.

Though I find several imbalances in my holistic assessment of her, it is Aiswarya's paradoxical breathing that I target first. I ask her to lie down over a special pranayama bolster I'd brought from the States. It about five inches wide and when you place it under the spine, the ribs on either side in the back are free to move unencumbered by any contact with the floor.

I ask her to place one hand on her belly and to breathe. This is an easy way to promote abdominal breathing, without having to think about it. I tell her to contract the abdominal muscles on the exhalation, progressively moving the belly in toward the spine.

Eyes closed, she goes inside and tries to allow the breath to happen spontaneously. It's almost as if the breath breathes you, I say. Within a few minutes her belly is reliably rising with the inhalation and falling with the exhalation. Her face looks more relaxed, and there's less tension around the eyes and mouth. I recommend that she breathe this way for five minutes a day. To this I add five minutes of simple asana, also employing healthy abdominal breathing.

This morning an email arrives asking me to teach at a symposium on integrative medicine at Harvard Medical School. The theme for the 2018 conference is Yoga and Ayurveda for Cancer. None of the organizers knows anything about my diagnosis or that I'm currently in India undergoing Ayurvedic treatments. I think, *You could not make this stuff up.*

From my bedroom window, I spot Amrutha hanging from a tree branch in the yard. She can just reach it wearing shoes with a low heel. I had never seen those before. Almost everyone here, male and female, wears flat chappals.

At breakfast I ask her what she was doing. "Push up," she says.

"Were you doing it for exercise? For fun?" She looks confused. "Were you hanging for enjoyment?"

"For getting taller." She is tiny, the shortest member of a short family. Now 15, Amrutha weighs only 29 kilos, about 64 pounds. She's picky about what she eats, refusing most vegetables and sweets. Many times, for the lunch she brings to school, she shovels a decent scoop of rice into her steel tiffin. Then with the precision of a lab scientist, she skims a spoonful of curry sauce from the bowl, being careful to avoid all vegetables, though a stray garbanzo doesn't bother her. To that she'll add a spoonful of what I call "blowtorch pickle condiment."

I've been attributing her small size to the fact that she was subsisting almost entirely on rice. At my suggestion, the family began feeding her more fish recently, which she had told me she liked. Already she is looking healthier. She says she's gained a kilo.

"By the way, this," I say, aping pulling myself up with arms overhead, "is called a pull-up." Dropping to the floor, I add, "This is a push up."

Then I say, "Can I tell you a secret?" She nods. "Hanging by your arms won't make you taller. Eating more good food, more curries, more vegetables, more fish, will make you grow."

Amrutha's English is not great, and my Malayalam is pathetic, but we've had a mostly unspoken connection since she was a little girl. With and without words, we communicate what we want to say to each other.

Aiswarya walks up the path returning from her course. I've been meaning to follow up with her on the yoga therapy we'd done.

"How is your breathing going?"

Fine, she says. As she speaks, I can see her releasing her belly and pulling it in as she inhales.

"Really?" I say. "Because that was a perfect paradoxical breath you just took."

I ask if she's been practicing. She has not.

"Can you spend a minute with me on the bench?"

Sitting side-by-side, I ask her to put one hand on her belly. "Feel the belly moving in toward the spine as you exhale. Feel your belly expanding as you inhale." I have her repeat this pattern for several more breaths.

"I'd like you to practice this for one minute a day. Can you do that?" She smiles, and says, "Of course."

I think she is surprised at how little I'm asking for. When I work with people therapeutically, I've found that the most important thing is to get them to practice every day, even if just a little. That's what starts to build the new neural pathways that pave the way for new habit patterns. The 10-minute practice I'd given her before was too ambitious, especially with her exam coming soon, and she hadn't been able to do it. I think I overshot.

My idea is that if she creates the foundation for a new habit, even if it's just for a minute a day, we can always build on it later. I teach my students that doing something every day is the key to inducing enduring neuroplastic change. If you're shooting for only one minute a day, and you end up doing 10, that's great. But that does not mean that the next day you can skip your practice. There are no "rollover" minutes. The dailiness of the repetition is what matters most.

One day during Nadi Shodhana pranayama, I notice without planning to that I've slowed my mantra down — and with it, the length of each breath. I'd guess that I'm breathing about once per minute, and I can sense that my body is indicating that it is ready for longer breath holding than I'd been doing.

The next morning, I try increasing the duration of each section of the breath during Nadi Shodhana — inhale, hold, exhale, hold — to 16 seconds. That's one breath every 64 seconds. It's challenging but doable, and it becomes my daily practice.

Slowly the breath like this feels like it's contributing to the heightened sense of groundedness I'm feeling in my physical body. It's calmed my vata. And I think it's been vital in helping to ratchet down my nervous system's twitchiness to normal (or close to normal) levels.

Less than a month before I left for this trip to India, I'd written a post on a popular yoga blog criticizing Dr. James Hamblin's assertion in *The Atlantic* that alternate nostril breathing is nothing more than a placebo. The irony is that when I wrote my critique of his article, I had no idea that Nadi Shodhana was about to become so important — not just to recovering from my cancer treatment — but to addressing my life-long Ayurvedic and nervous system imbalances. The time I've spent on my daily asana and meditation practice has certainly benefited me during this trip, but my guess is that it's the breathwork that's been most important. And it keeps getting deeper.

―――――――

Resting these final three weeks before flying to England, I feel my strength increasing. I've balanced myself Ayurvedically for the first time in my life, and for three months now, it has lasted. I feel grounded and calm like never before. My injured leg has been completely rehabilitated. The combination of the MFR, yoga, and Krishna's treatments has rendered my spine more pliable than it was before I got sick. And fasting feels like an important addition to my toolkit. It helped me get through chemo, and is doing, I suspect, much more. Rather than feeling like a burden, discovering fasting feels like another silver lining of what I've endured.

My yoga practice is becoming stronger. I'm even doing the occasional handstand, which due to shoulder problems and then the cancer, I hadn't done for three years.

And with no more restrictions on exercise from Krishna, I've returned to dancing. I'd danced some down south, and started getting more energetic about it in Vermont. But now I'm stepping it up.

I have a mix I've been evolving over the years, rotating songs in and out, mostly funky and soulful African-American tunes of the last 50 years, but pretty eclectic. "Let It Whip." "Thank You (Falettinme Be Mice Elf Agin)." "Boogie On Reggae Woman." "Mambo Yo Yo." "I Can't Get Next to You." "What Goes Around...Comes Around." "Uptown Funk." Pharrell Williams' "Happy." Amos Lee's "Dreamin'." And lately, in heavy rotation, "Where Is the Love?"

I've been dancing by myself at home for fun and exercise my entire adult life, but how I move has changed a lot. At 18, at parties and clubs, it was about trying to find the beat and not look stupid. Even as I improved, the focus was always on outward appearances. Years ago, I decided all mirrors had to go from the room I danced in at home to shift the focus to the bodily experience. The softer, breath-centered yoga I've been doing the last few years, as well as the chi gung, have had a big effect on how I move to some of the same songs I danced to way back when.

Now, standing in a semi-squatting position not unlike Goddess pose, I carve the air with my hands, aware of the flow of prana, as in Tai Chi. I try to inhabit the music, feeling the emotion and love the artists put into it and to translate that to my body. My awareness of chaining through the myofascia connects my lower abdomen and the flow of the breath to movements of my arm and legs.

With slow, mindful breathing, the nervous system stays calm even with maximal effort. No matter how fast and hard I dance now, how much I move my arms or kick up my legs, no matter how high my heart rate climbs, I discover that I never exceed six or seven slow, smooth breaths per minute. From an Ayurvedic perspective there's more earth and water in my dance. I always had the fire and air.

More and more, I am letting my body tell me where to go and what to move, instead of — as I always did before — using my mind to plan some movement that I'd task my body to carry out. This movement is analogous to the myofascial release practice of "unwinding," which is believed to help relieve fascial restrictions. Now I dance from the inside out.

Aiswarya is playing a song on her phone, which I can tell is her singing. She has a sweet voice, and often sings along with songs on the radio. Occasionally, she chants in the prayer room. The song she's playing sounds like the Hindi east/west mashes on the station she listens to, halfway between modern-day R&B and Indian pop with its lilting vocal inflections.

"Is that a famous singer?" I ask.

"I wrote this," she says. It isn't finished and she doesn't have all the words yet.

"What is it about?"

"A girl is looking for something."

"Is it a love song?"

"I think so."

I don't believe, as some yogis do, that before we are born our soul chooses our parents. But I like this concept as a metaphor. Why would a son choose Hurricane Betty as his mother? And why Pop, from whom seldom was heard an encouraging word?

It was Pop who pushed me into studying medicine. If he hadn't had this agenda for my life, I would probably have chosen another path. But I think my journey through medicine has served me well. My years of medical practice taught me what it is to be a clinician and not just a theoretician, and that serves me well in my yoga therapy work to this day. My medical training was also hugely important in my recent adventures as a patient.

Whatever the limitations of Pop's intellectually rigorous — yet emotionally and spiritually impoverished — take on psychology, I grew up in an environment where understanding the mind was valued. Studying the mind is the central preoccupation of classical yoga, as described by Patanjali in his seminal *Yoga Sutras*. My father modeled intellectual rigor, and precision in language, and he expected these from us. And, of course, his needing me to achieve on the tennis court was what led me to yoga — though I wouldn't figure that out for quite some time. As difficult a guru as Pop was for me, and as much as I suffered under his tutelage, to carry out my dharma of writing and teaching and exploring the body and the mind, I couldn't have done much better.

As for my mother — if my bond to her had been stronger, if she'd been able to figure out what her little kid needed, if she'd been capable of showering love on the helpless being that arrived in her life — I might have been happy to simply coast in adulthood. Instead, I gave up my medical practice and embarked on the path of yoga. Without all the suffering I'd had in my early years, which in turn begot still more suffering, I don't think I would have been motivated to choose that less-traveled path. Suffering is universal, and people react to it differently, but I think my early-life trauma is what drew me to spirituality.

From Mom, the master of projects, I also learned organization. Neither of my brothers got this piece. She was practical in a way that Pop, who called himself the "absent-minded professor," was not. He had trouble opening a box of Grape Nuts without destroying the lid.

Mom was smart about money, Pop was not. Again and again, she figured ways that our family could have a high standard of living, on much less income than you might suppose would be necessary. I've done the same for years. Due to the money smarts I got from Mom, I've been able to follow my interests wherever they've taken me — including to India for months on end, on multiple occasions. When I needed to pay for my cancer care, I was able to take funds out of my retirement savings — only possible because I've been parking away 10 percent of my never-that-high income since my 20s. But unlike Mom, I have yet to figure out how to make houses magically appear.

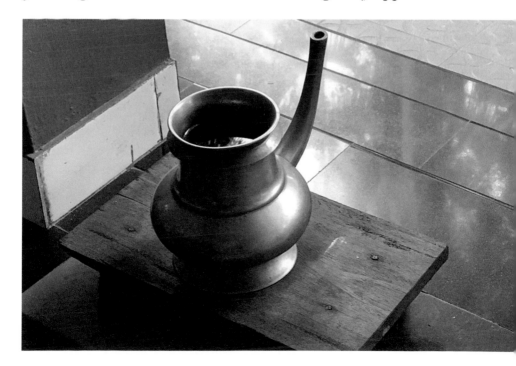

Out for a late morning walk, I am thinking about Tony. In some ways, our relationship has not been easy. I'd always thought it was because we are so different. He's more conventional, more socially conservative than I am. But I realize it can't be just that, as I have several close friends who are more traditional than he is.

Growing up, Tony played by the rules and I broke them. It occurs to me that it must have been infuriating for him that I always seemed to get away with it. It's as if he were the older brother of the prodigal son, who had to watch his wayward sibling welcomed home with all forgiven. His karma was to be the good kid with a couple of parents who valued nonconformity at least as much as success.

Tony is brilliant and has a ton of pitta. That same fierceness I experienced from him on the tennis court, he's applied to medicine and his research. My big brother is a slightly nerdy brainiac, an academic heavy hitter, the holder of an endowed chair at a top medical school, the vice president of his national specialty organization. He's been awarded millions of dollars in NIH research grants. Not many professors in his position — even some with exalted reputations — are also top-flight clinicians.

I've thought that he's a great doctor since I was a medical resident, when we were both living in Boston. This was confirmed for me just before he moved north for Madelyn's job. In his last days at the diabetes clinic, patient after patient told him how much his care had meant to them. Some were in tears. Tony is not a man who shows a lot of emotion, but he was visibly moved when he told us about these conversations at dinner.

In the hyper-competitive world of academic medicine — populated by people who strut around hospital wards like the rooster in Krishna's yard — Tony stands out as a mensch. He's friendly. Humble. Soft-spoken. He tries to connect with his patients. When I contemplate all these qualities, the closest match I can find is Dr. Jeremiah Clark, the radiation oncologist, to whom I will always feel indebted.

Ironically, both of us being doctors probably made relating harder for Tony and me — our intellectual differences activated that old competitive groove. We had different worldviews before medicine, and they affect how we view doctoring to this day. He wears bow ties to work — and I wear mala beads.

I think back to the way Pop pitted us against each other in tennis, the constant verbal one-upmanship at the dinner table, Pop's telling him that I was the real scholar in the family. I contemplate my failure to fly in and help him after he ruptured both quadriceps tendons. Yes, it would have been inconvenient, but that's a lousy excuse.

A realization hits me like a blow across the chest. Despite my efforts to feel love flowing in and out over the last decade, I realize that my heart has never fully opened to Tony. I've felt judged by him and in return I've judged him. Old resentments have kept a wall between us. I burst into tears.

I let the tears stream down my face as I walk the public road, not bothering to wipe them away, and thankfully I encounter no one. I need to call Tony and talk this through. It is the last thing I feel like doing, but I know it is necessary. And it's exactly the tough medicine I prescribe to my yoga students.

When there's something not quite right in a relationship — say a vibrant friendship feels like it's changing for the worse — the counterintuitive and necessary step is to initiate a conversation about it. And this has been borne out by my life experience. I've had these difficult conversations with both Tomas and Andy. In each case we came out the other side with our relationship not just repaired, but made stronger by the trust and confidence that comes with speaking from your heart, and having it received well.

———————

I call Tony. I time it so that I can catch him after Madelyn has left for work. I tell him that I'd been thinking about the way Pop pitted us against each other in tennis, and how excruciating I found those matches.

"I have some memory of that," he says. "He pitted all of us against each other." I knew that was his experience, but I'd never felt pitted against Ray. The thirteen-year age difference between us was enough to eliminate any sibling rivalry.

"Ray told me that Pop said at your PhD graduation that I was 'the real scholar in the family.'"

"Yep. Pop said that."

I apologize again for not coming to help him when he was rehabbing after his quad tendon ruptures. "I feel terrible about that." He is gracious, as he'd been the first time I'd said how sorry I was.

"I was thinking that it could not have been easy being my big brother. You were a good kid who did everything expected of him. I broke all the rules, and got away with it."

"Mom used to say that you could walk through walls," Tony says. I was legendary in the family for getting permission that normally wasn't granted, as when I'd convinced my high school French teacher to allow me to skip class and study independently. "But sometimes you also walked through people."

Tony has likely harbored that sentiment for decades, but this is the first I've ever heard it. We are being honest with each other in a way we've never done before. We speak for perhaps 45 minutes. To my mind, it is the best conversation we've ever had.

Toward the end of the conversation, I describe how great and highly functional Krishna's family is; how much I feel like I'm part of it.

"It's easier," Tony says, "because they are not *actually* your family." Can't argue with that.

————————

After a coconut sits in the sun for about four months, a foamy growth fills its insides. Krishna shows me one, cut open to reveal the filling. Bindu takes it to the kitchen and cuts it into bite-sized chunks and serves it to me at the table. It's airy, crunchy, slightly wet, with a hint of sweet coconut taste.

Across the table, Krishna piles his plate with tapioca, looking like boiled potatoes, and then spoons on a white condiment, flecked with bits of green.

"Is that coconut chutney?" I ask — a condiment I love. It is. "Is it made from mature coconut?"

"Yes," he says, "and some green chilies, a small onion, and salt. You can add a little coconut oil for a nice taste."

I'd been avoiding the starchy tapioca due to my concerns with carbohydrates fueling cancer, but I want to try it. I fish a chuck from the pot. Krishna warns me the chutney is spicy, but I think it will be okay. I pick out one filament of green chili from the spoonful I've taken, just in case, and plaster the remainder on the side of the tapioca.

It hits my tongue and the combination of the starch and the chutney elicit a deep release in my nervous system. It's like inhaling a whiff of the head oil or massaging the third eye in Dhara. Whatever my thoughts were about carbs potentially fueling cancer, at this moment my body does not seem to be the least bit concerned.

I didn't choose this cancer adventure. In trying to deal with it skillfully, I did the best I could, given the necessarily incomplete and often conflicting information I'd amassed by the time each decision needed to be made. And overall, I'm happy with my choices.

I felt a twinge of regret when I learned about the metabolic theory of cancer, after my treatments were already completed. Early on during chemoradiation, I briefly swished and swallowed the amino acid, L-Glutamine. I'd found some evidence that the dietary supplement — one of the only alternative reductionist tools I wound up using — could reduce the risk of radiation mucositis, the painful ulceration of the lining of the mouth and throat. But when I later read about the metabolic theory of cancer, I learned that other than sugar, glutamine is cancer's preferred fuel. But given the fasting I did, and the amount of time I spent in ketosis during my treatments, I doubt the glutamine did too much harm.

Throughout my illness I chose the path of holism, taking one small step at a time, trying to address many different aspects of my situation in hope of moving the whole in a helpful direction. I addressed my structure and my physiology, my breathing, my nervous system, as well as my mind, my emotions, and my spirit.

Through an examination of my past, and of my relationships with family, friends, and lovers, I continued my journey of psychological excavation, jettisoning attitudes and behaviors that may have served me in my difficult childhood, but which are no longer needed.

Through the steady practice of trying to feel the love of the Mother, over the last decade I have re-patterned my neural architecture in a way I wasn't sure was even possible. Now I can also feel the love, stunted and blocked as it may have been, of my own mother. Imbued with the feeling of being cherished and protected, I no longer need, as I once did, a steady dose of attention to feel okay about myself.

I've come into balance Ayurvedically for the first time in my life, and I've managed to maintain this balance for three months. With my vata now under control, I have embodied the kapha that was always my birthright, but which was never expressed. My kapha nature was buried beneath an avalanche of vata, which is the opposite of kapha in nearly every respect. Vata is lighter, quicker, more irregular, less stable. My kapha was so obscured in the swirl of activity with which I surrounded myself, and the workings of my endlessly busy mind that it evaded my notice for years. As far as I know, only Chandukutty Vaidyar picked up on it.

All those years of vata derangement caused another problem: they depleted my body of ojas (OH-juss). Ojas is the healthy aspect of kapha, and it's linked to immune function and contentment. Mine was depleted from a life of the drying wind of vata blowing on the body's watery goodness. When I got to India, Krishna judged my ojas level to be 60 percent of normal, which is not terrible but not ideal. That was likely a big improvement from what it had been at the end of chemoradiation.

A month after he began treating me, Krishna assessed my ojas level at 70 percent. To measure my level, he didn't touch me or even move — he just paused a moment, and reported the result. What was interesting was that his assessments matched my own. He appeared to just know — it seemed that he'd inherited at least a little bit of Chandukutty's magic. I gauged the ojas level by putting my fingers on my wrist, as I did every morning, but I've never been able to just look at someone and know how much ojas they've got.

Two months into this trip, my pulse exams revealed that my ojas had continued to trend higher, so I asked him to reassess. After pondering it for a moment, he said "80 percent," which was exactly what I'd been thinking. Toward the end of my stay, my ojas level had risen to somewhere between 80 and 90 percent of normal. Krishna told me he had never seen that much ojas in any patient he'd ever treated.

I'm grounded now. My voice is deeper. I wake more slowly, and move more deliberately. I'm less fearful. Love flows in and out like never before. Kapha. Earth and water. The two elements that constitute sweetness, according to Ayurveda — both in foods and in emotions.

While you could call what I've done an example of integrative medicine, typically defined as the combination of conventional and alternative medical therapies, I view it through the lens of holism and reductionism. My modus operandi was to devise — and constantly modify as conditions warranted — a comprehensive holistic plan addressing every aspect of mind, body, spirit, and environment. To this, I selectively added the reductionist tools I thought most likely to be helpful, like radiation therapy, the Cisplatin chemo, ibuprofen, narcotic pain relievers, and the shingles vaccine.

This could be a model for healthcare in the future. The foundation would be holistic approaches to prevention and treatment — at least in those individuals willing to take on the work they often demand. Reductionist measures like drugs, surgery, and dietary supplements could be the complementary or adjunctive care, employed only when dietary, lifestyle, and holistic treatment modalities don't suffice.

———————

As hard as I've worked to get through the challenge of cancer, I have also surrendered the illusion that I can control it. Optimistic as I am, I am aware that my efforts may not have been enough. Part of my hopefulness is that I know that if the cancer should recur, I have many tools to help me get through it. To heal even if I cannot be cured. To live however much life I have left with joy and contentment and love. And with the urgency the diagnosis has brought, I am determined to live life more fully, to bring even more passion and discipline to the work I feel like I've been put on the planet to do.

This is not a tale of my efforts to get back to normal — back to life as it was before I had cancer. I aimed higher than that. It's about how I used the challenges the diagnosis presented to live my life more authentically, in a more balanced way, one better aligned with my life's purpose.

Was getting cancer a good thing? Could it possibly be the best thing that's ever happened to me? It might have killed me, and still could. But my life is better today than the day I was diagnosed, whether I'm cured or not. It's not even a close contest. Big chunks of what's better might not have happened otherwise.

I will continue to play the hand I'm dealt as skillfully as I can. As a kid at the lake house, playing the card game Hearts with Mom and Pop and Debbie on rainy summer days, I was always looking to "shoot the moon." Some things don't change.

It's amazing how this place, this land, is sinking into me, and I am sinking into it. I mean that literally, because as my nervous system has relaxed, the tissues on my feet and legs have opened, now cupping the earth as never before. According to the *Hatha Yoga Pradipika*, Nadi Shodhana can make your legs feel rooted like the trunks of trees. I am both more grounded, and from that rootedness, I am able to extend upwards with greater ease.

I'm not saying that I want to live in Kerala full time, just that it feels like home, like somewhere I belong. Even though I believe that my work is in the west, I feel the love in this land. I can inhale its healing energy. As I think about the subzero winter temperatures back in Burlington, I find myself fantasizing about coming here for a few months every year to recharge, to create, to heal, to rest, to imbibe its shakti, and to recharge mine.

My deepening friendship with Krishna has been a highlight of this trip. It's so easy and natural, and there's a trust and an understanding we've built over years. Second only to my relationship with Krishna has been the one with Aiswarya. Between her test preparation course and our many conversations, she's probably spoken more English in the last four months than in her entire life. Her dramatically improved English allowed us to have dozens of meaningful talks this trip, and hundreds of fun interactions. I've had the latter with Amrutha as well, but only a couple of good talks. The language barrier has stopped me from conversing much with other family members, but I still feel connected to them.

It occurs to me that Aiswarya, the good kid who wins

all the academic prizes, has embodied the same evolutionary niche as Tony. And Amrutha, who breaks all the rules and gets away with it, is a rebel like me.

———————

Sanyasi is the fourth and final stage in life as described by ancient Indian texts. It is the stage to seek moksha, spiritual liberation, whether attainable in this lifetime or not. Some monks skip right to this phase, bypassing marriage and a regular job. But for most Hindus, the idea is that first you go to school, then you turn to a career, have a family, and, only after your responsibilities to your work and children have been met, do you renounce the world and go meditate in some forest or cave.

I call what I'm doing "monk mode," but I haven't gone quite that far. My cave is in a comfortable apartment in a beautiful town. I work in the world intermittently, and I find it fulfilling. I eat sumptuous, high prana food. I have satisfying friendships and, among my friends, family, and fellow yogis, a sense of community. My ability to schedule my time as I wish allows me to practice more yoga than most people could, even if they wanted to — and the practice is a continual source of discovery and joy.

———————

As I meditate on the platform in the back of the temple, I gently engage Mula Bandha, the root lock, lightly contracting the muscles of the pelvic floor above the perineum. Doing this provides a stable foundation that allows the breath to flow effortlessly in and out.

The air is redolent with the fragrance of coconut husks that smolder in the fire pit beside me. I used to recite the Durga mantra silently — that is, without voicing it out loud. Now, after years of practice, it's as if my mind never quite stops reverberating with the echo of thousands of repetitions. Rather than say the mantra, I get quiet and I listen for it. The sounds resonate in my consciousness, and I feel the love of the Mother. As I focus my attention on the area between my navel and solar plexus, I feel a subtle energy lifting from Muladhara. It travels up through each successive chakra, all the way to Sahasrara, at the crown of my head — connecting all these chakras like beads on a thread. If I were to lift too strongly, that energetic filament would break. If I didn't lift strongly enough, the thread would sag like a loose guitar string. I aim to find a middle path between effort and ease — in my practice and in my life.

As I sit, my knees sink into the platform. My pelvis grounds solidly into the block beneath my hips, which I brought with me to the temple. For most of my life, the airy nature of vata meant my energy was directed upwards, almost as if I were levitating. Now, sitting on this holy ground, I feel connected to the earth.

Bead by bead, the mala passes between my thumb and middle finger. The larger guru bead, which hangs at the bottom when I wear the mala, marks each round. I come to it three times before I loop the strand back around my neck and cross my hands over my heart. Feeling the emotion evoked by this hand position, Hridaya Mudra, I silently repeat my sankalpa: *I am feeling loved, protected, nourished, and cherished by the Mother.* I rest floating in this watery energy, and it supports me like the soft swell of the sea.

With each inhalation I hear the mantra, and imagine all the shakti of this sacred place — the pujas, the prayers, the luscious nature all around — coming into my heart along with the love of the Mother. As I exhale, I visualize the healing energy of the Mother's love flowing throughout my body. My mouth and neck, still recovering from the chemoradiation that ended almost 12 months ago, are bathed in love.

After a few breaths, I expand the sphere of my awareness beyond myself, until it includes the temple and everyone in it. Next, I imagine sending that love farther and farther out until it envelops the entire planet, and then the universe.

As I walk along the side of the road, heading home from the temple, I feel a sense of fullness. Not ecstasy, but a kind of abiding tranquility. I remember myself at 14, lying in the woods by the lake house, near the edge of the water, staring up at the underside of a sugar maple. There was something I was searching for but couldn't name. If I could have willed it into being, I would have.

And then I understand: *This is it*. It was there back then, too. The Mother, the universe, the God, whatever you want to call it, was nourishing and protecting me all those years I felt adrift. I just couldn't feel it.

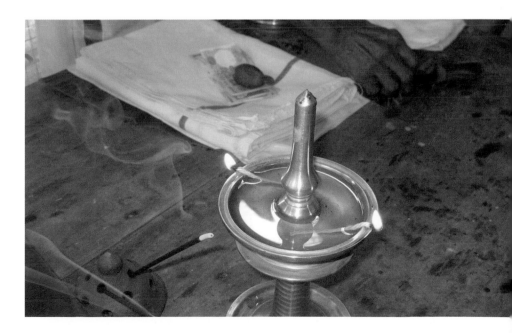

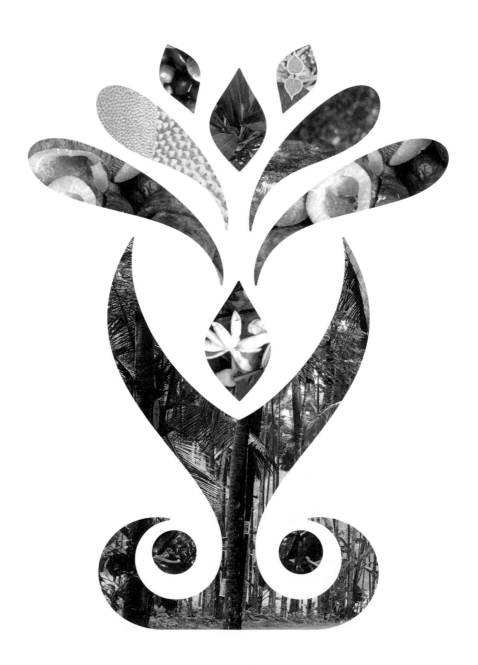

EPILOGUE

It's been three months since I left Kerala. I am about to give a plenary address at the annual conference of the International Association of Yoga Therapists (IAYT) in the ballroom of a Washington-area hotel. Dr. Dilip Sarkar introduces me. He's a retired surgeon, and the organization's outgoing president. His praise is over the top — I'm actually a little embarrassed. I had already decided that this was the right occasion to go public with my cancer diagnosis, but Dilip beats me to the punch. I hadn't expected that, but I'm fine with it.

For a variety of reasons, when I needed to undergo chemotherapy and radiation at the beginning of last year, I opted to keep it private. While I'm sure my yoga friends and colleagues would have been supportive, I decided not to say anything. I shared my situation only with an intimate group of friends and family. In retrospect, I think I made the right call.

Before the conference, I had another visit with Dr. Kuantai, the ENT specialist in Burlington. She thought everything looked great. My body weight was back to normal. My strength and stamina were better than ever.

The vata derangement I've had since infancy hadn't reappeared, even with transcontinental flights and a hectic teaching schedule in London.

I do have less saliva than I used to, I told Dr. Kuantai, but I make sure to drink more fluids with meals, which softens and moistens the food. I've also come up with a little trick, which no doctor has ever mentioned: Whenever my mouth feels dry, I chew some gum, and immediately it stimulates my damaged salivary glands — problem solved. I think of it as a three-pronged training program for my mouth: mastication for the jaw muscles, swallowing for the throat, and saliva generation for the glands.

My appointment with Dr. Kuantai happened to coincide with one of my water fasts. "I haven't eaten anything for three days," I told her. She was amazed that I looked so good. I'd decided to try a four-day fast with each change of season, and spring had sprung in Vermont. Ayurveda suggests that the seasonal change is a good time for a brief fast, especially in the spring. I explained to her that I was planning on following each quarterly fast with three days of a high fat, low-carb, moderate protein diet. The goal was to keep myself in ketosis longer, potentially boosting the anti-cancer effect. Last summer, the four-day water fast was in some ways stressful, and my sleep was fitful. This time, one year after the end of treatment, my nervous system seemed unperturbed by the lack of food, and I had been sleeping well.

I've decided against going on a ketogenic diet full-time, even though many are now recommending it for cancer. I don't want to have to buy an electronic scale, don't want to have to weigh every single ingredient I cook with, and measure the exact quantities of carbohydrates and proteins I take in. Many people do it, but it doesn't feel like something I want or need to do right now. Plus, the books I've read say the diet is nearly impossible for a vegetarian, which I am (except for the occasional piece of fish). My hunch is that the fasting is actually the most effective piece of the puzzle anyway.

I'm also not convinced it's a good idea to give up all the prana of the fresh vegetables, fruits, and whole grains that a ketogenic diet would deprive me of. I still eat complex carbohydrates though I've cut the quantity to some degree. I've already given up white rice, potatoes, and refined grains as well as some fruits particularly high in sugar. Last summer I gave up all foods containing refined sugar: chocolate, desserts, honey, and my beloved maple syrup. Maple sugar candy, molded into the shape of the tree's leaves, was like crack for me when I was a toddler.

It's shocking how little I miss any of it. I've jettisoned my beloved dark chocolate, but I still get to use organic cacao, which is unsweetened. I add it to the herbal chai I make most mornings at home. I've also decided to keep drinking the beautiful full-fat raw milk I get in Burlington. It's the best milk I've ever had. It adds natural sweetness to the chai, and because I drink it Ayurvedic style, warmed just until little bubbles appear, the lack of pasteurization poses no risk. While some say milk could accelerate the growth of any cancer cells that remain in my body, my gut tells me it's not going to kill me.

I don't want to go keto full time, but I do plan to follow the diet for three days after each water fast. There are enough vegetarian options to make this doable. This way I should be able to stay in ketosis for almost a week straight. This should promote autophagy, giving my immune system a reboot. I also plan to continue my practice of fasting for 15 hours every night between dinner and breakfast.

Unlike most of my doctors down south, Dr. Kuantai seemed fascinated by the holistic approaches I'm employing. She seemed particularly intrigued by the mouth work I do on myself, and sometimes receive, which is designed to release fascial adhesions. She said, "I always learn so much from your visits."

Dr. Kuantai's openness may be a function of her youth. The only other physician who had seemed supportive of my integrative approach, Dr. Mitchell, the oncology fellow who was working with Dr. Shanahan, was also young. "Whatever you're doing," she said at the end of the appointment, "keep on doing it."

My experience as a yoga therapist is that not many older physicians embrace it, except for the few who are already yoga practitioners. Getting older doctors, including leaders of the field, to accept a new way of thinking — or in the case of holism, a very old way of thinking — isn't easy. The medical profession is beginning to show more interest in holistic medicine. This is less because doctors are changing their minds, though, and more because doctors with older ideas are retiring, and being replaced by a new generation.

Change is afoot, and not only in the US. While I was in England, I was invited to speak at a hearing in the House of Lords in Westminster. I chose to discuss the healing benefits of yoga. It's on such occasions that yoga research proves most useful: Every week there are more citable studies to choose from. For example, a research professor who also addressed the Lords that day mentioned studies that have found that patients who do yoga have lower health care costs — music to any politician's ears.

At the end of the session, the Parliamentarians established an All-Party Parliamentary Group focused on yoga. This was the first time any legislature, anywhere, had ever taken such a step. The Group's mission is to bring more yoga into Britain's National Health Service, and into British society in general. Not only patients are being targeted; the project also aims to bring the benefits of yoga to the stressed-out health care workers of the chronically underfunded NHS.

And there's good news from Kerala: Aiswarya had just received her big test results, and she did well. Krishna would later tell me that she landed a spot at one of the country's top Ayurvedic medical colleges. She'll start soon. I am so proud of her. She'll get her medical license, but will continue to be exposed to more traditional Malabar-style Ayurveda, through Krishna and other mentors he'll help her find.

All this is in my mind as I take the stage at the IAYT conference and give my plenary address. My talk receives a raucous standing ovation (full disclosure: many at this year's gathering have received standing ovations). As the applause dies down, the organization's incoming president, Dr. Amy Wheeler, asks the audience to close their eyes and direct healing energy to me. The room goes silent. I soak it in, placing both palms, crossed, over my heart. Then I join the group as we chant a powerful Om. The crowded hotel ballroom brims over with love and support.

Amy and I met for the first time at dinner the night before. A group of us, wanting to escape the air-conditioned hotel, had walked to a restaurant with an outdoor terrace. I felt an immediate bond with her. Pitta-kapha types have been entering my life more and more in recent years. My guess is that Amy, driven and loving, is among them. As a college student, she told me, she'd been a serious athlete, competing in the Heptathlon. With her strong shoulders and arms, she could undoubtedly launch a shot put much farther than I could.

After the conference has adjourned, I spot Amy sitting with Dilip and other members of the IAYT board at a table in the hotel lobby. I stop to say goodbye. Looking into her eyes, I see a familiar maternal sweetness. I realize she reminds me of my friends Theresa and Linda, who provided the model of motherly love that served me so well in my healing journey.

I say to her, "You are such a love bunny."

She pauses, looking at me, her eyes both kind and discerning. "It's amazing," she says. "Your heart is completely open."

That, I tell her, is a whole other story.

ACKNOWLEDGEMENTS

There are more people who have helped me on this journey than I can name here. You know who you are. Let me mention just a few.

My healing from cancer and its treatment was facilitated by the love and help of friends and family. Loved ones took me into their homes, into their hearts and into their prayers. Tony, and especially my sister-in-law Madelyn, supported me during my cancer care in more ways than I can count. Madelyn has been a font of sage sisterly advice for years. My sister Debbie, too, was generous to a fault, and was prepared to do more had I needed it. My friends Andy and Tomas were always there for me. Mark and Linda did so much to ease my transition back to Vermont. I have no doubt that all this love and support made all the healing approaches I used more effective.

I am indebted, of course, to the many fine physicians and other health care professionals I encountered during this journey, as well as the many holistic healers. It was my great fortune to wind up under the care of the extraordinary doctor I've called Jeremiah Clark in this book. Ginny Jurken made a huge contribution to my rehabilitation after treatment, and has been a great friend and supporter the whole way. Krishna Dasan and his family, and everyone at Kallyani Ayurveda in Kerala, must have been sent by the God.

On my path in yoga, there were two teachers with whom I worked the longest, week-in and week-out, to whom I am particularly indebted. I will be forever grateful to Patricia Walden, who first opened the door to yoga for me, both personally and professionally. Her grace, her generous teaching, and her obvious love of the practice were what drew me in, but it may have been her playful sense of humor — which I only got to see once I knew her well — that sealed the deal. During my nine years in Berkeley and Oakland, I was thrilled to study with Donald Moyer. Many times, when I followed some new vein of awareness in my practice at home, I found myself exclaiming "Thank You, Donald!" And in Ayurveda, it was Chandukutty Vaidyar who appeared when I was ready for something more traditional, more authentic. He showed me that Ayurveda is an ocean as deep as yoga, as deep as modern science.

Many friends and colleagues looked at various drafts of the manuscript and offered editing suggestions. I am particularly grateful to my friends Amelia, Ginny and Vicki, and above all to my big brother Ray, who has always had my back. My friend William spent dozens of hours with me, poring over individual sentences — our work together made this book a better book, and me a better writer. My extraordinary editor Beth Rashbaum was so good on *Yoga as Medicine* that I hired her for this book, and she didn't disappoint. I am grateful to Keith Gordon for smart and gracious copy-editing. Big thanks to David Grotrian for painting the book cover I'd been envisioning, but having a hard time finding an artist to do. And Hallelujah for my amazing friend and designer Steph Salmon from Gotham City Graphics.

I couldn't have done this without you.

ABOUT THE AUTHOR

Timothy McCall, MD is a board-certified internist, Medical Editor of Yoga Journal since 2002, and author of the bestselling *Yoga as Medicine: The Yogic Prescription for Health and Healing* (Bantam). His first book was the critically acclaimed, *Examining Your Doctor: A Patient's Guide to Avoiding Harmful Medical Care* (Citadel Press). He serves on the editorial

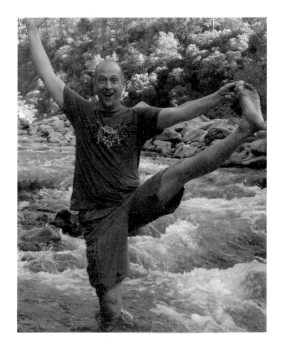

board of *The International Journal of Yoga Therapy*, and co-edited and contributed to the 2016 medical textbook, *The Principles and Practice of Yoga in Health Care* (Handspring Publishing).

Dr. McCall practiced medicine in the Boston area for a dozen years before devoting himself in the late 1990s to yoga therapy. He has studied yoga with BKS Iyengar and TKV Desikachar, and also with Patricia Walden, Rod Stryker, and Donald Moyer. He studied Ayurveda as an apprentice and patient of a traditional Ayurvedic doctor, Chandukutty Vaidyar, at his clinic in Kerala, India.

His articles have appeared in dozens of publications, including *The New England Journal of Medicine*, *JAMA*, *The Los Angeles Times* and *The Nation*. From 1996 to 2001, his medical commentaries were featured on the public radio program *Marketplace*. He has given numerous workshops and keynote addresses at conferences sponsored by the National Institutes of Health, Yoga Journal, the International Association of Yoga Therapists, and the Smithsonian Institution.

Timothy is the founder and director of the Yoga As Medicine® Seminars and Teacher Trainings. He lives in Burlington, Vermont and lectures and teaches around the world. Learn more at www.DrMcCall.com.

INDEX

PRAISE FOR "YOGA AS MEDICINE"

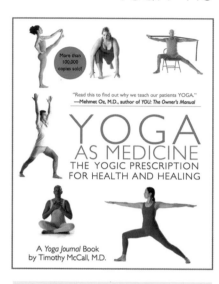

"If you care about your body and want to learn to listen more carefully to its messages, and to take good care of it over the long haul, you will find this book a godsend, whether you are young or old, firm or infirm, a new-comer to yoga or an old-timer. It is the first comprehensive medical look at the benefits of yoga and its therapeutic uses. Timothy McCall has done a great service to the field of mind/body medicine."

— Jon Kabat-Zinn, PhD,
Professor of Medicine emeritus,
University of Massachusetts
Medical School,
author of *Wherever You Go,
There You Are*

"*Yoga as Medicine* is a powerfully clear, accessible and practical guide to creating a vibrantly healthy body, mind, and spirit. What a tremendous contribution to healing and human potential!"

— Joan Borysenko, PhD,
author of *Minding the Body,
Mending the Mind*

"Yoga *is* medicine. Dr. McCall shows us, step by step, with helpful pictures, clear prescriptions, and up-to-date references, how it's practiced, and how it can help us to heal in body, mind, and spirit."

— James S. Gordon, MD,
Founder and Director,
The Center for Mind-Body
Medicine, author of *Manifesto for
a New Medicine*

"This is a landmark book. *Yoga as Medicine provides* a remarkable perspective on the breadth and depth of Yoga therapy, and many leading practitioners, both in the West and India, in a uniquely educational, engaging, and inspiring way."

— John Kepner,
   Executive Director,
   International Association of Yoga
   Therapists

"Timothy McCall skillfully introduces us into the vast universe of yogic healing, affording access to compelling new models of balance and wholeness for body, mind and spirit."

— Dr. David Frawley,
   author of *Yoga and Ayurveda*

"*Yoga as Medicine* is beautifully organized and presented, making it instantly readable and practical for anyone desiring better health or immediate help with a particular problem."

— Christiane Northrup, MD,
   author of *The Wisdom of Menopause*

"The next best thing to having the doctor right there beside you. An instant classic."

— Richard Rosen,
   author of *The Yoga of Breath*

"McCall's fine articulation of yoga's healing potential will appeal to a large audience of instructors, students, physicians and their patients."

— *Publishers Weekly*
   (Starred Review)

"Read this to find out why we teach our patients YOGA."

— Mehmet Oz, MD,
   Professor and Vice
   Chairman,
   NY Presbyterian/
   Columbia University
   Hospital and
   author of *You: The Owner's Manual*

PRAISE FOR
"THE PRINCIPLES AND PRACTICE OF YOGA IN HEALTH CARE"

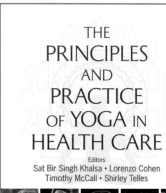

THE
PRINCIPLES
AND
PRACTICE
OF **YOGA** IN
HEALTH CARE

Editors
Sat Bir Singh Khalsa • Lorenzo Cohen
Timothy McCall • Shirley Telles

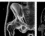 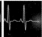

Forewords by
Dean Ornish, MD • Belle Monappa Hegde, MD, PhD, FRCP

HANDSPRING
PUBLISHING

"This is an extraordinary book. The authors have curated an extensive selection of research, providing the first state-of-the-art review of yoga therapy as an edited, scholarly, medically oriented textbook with a strong evidence-based focus on research and practice. There is strong representation internationally from both leading yoga researchers and yoga therapists."

– Dean Ornish, MD,
Founder and President,
Preventive Medicine Research
Institute, Clinical Professor
of Medicine, University of
California, San Francisco,
author of *Dr. Dean Ornish's
Program for Reversing Heart
Disease*

"The efforts of this group of researchers to put together a textbook of the yogic sciences is a timely contribution to bring yogic sciences to mainstream healing efforts. The many leading international yoga researchers who have contributed to this volume have presented the scientific rationale for yoga therapy and the existing published biomedical research evidence in a rigorous and comprehensive manner that will be appreciated by both conventional and integrative medicine researchers and clinicians, and the contribution of leading yoga therapists on practical clinical applications is invaluable. Given that this is the first textbook of its kind, it fills an important need, and will therefore serve a significant role for health care and healing in modern society."

— Professor Belle Monappa Hegde MD, PhD, FRCP
 Padma Bhushan Awardee 2010
 Cardiologist & Former Vice Chancellor
 Manipal University, India

"As health professionals, yoga therapist, and practitioners of yoga consider how to integrate yoga into healthcare, there is a need to evaluate and compile the yoga literature to date. This book...fulfills this need by sifting through published studies and producing an impressive medical textbook and reference on yoga therapy. Numerous authors from the fields of research and yoga therapy contributed their expertise in creating a compendium of yoga as applied to healthcare.

This is the first medically oriented textbook of yoga that comprehensively reviews the scientific literature of yoga for healthcare. It will be the standard reference for medical evidence of yoga therapy. Yoga therapy and research continues to grow, and this book presents the culmination and impact of yoga therapy today."

— Gurjeet S. Birdee, M.D., M.P.H.
 Assistant Professor of Internal Medicine, Pediatrics
 Vanderbilt University Medical Center

PRAISE FOR "EXAMINING YOUR DOCTOR"

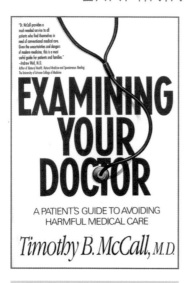

"This is one of the few books of its genre that I can warmly recommend to the general public. It is honest, well-informed, and full of good, sensible advice."
— Arnold S. Relman, MD,
   Harvard Medical School,
   Emeritus Editor-in-Chief,
   The New England Journal of Medicine

"Frank, provocative, and comprehensive, this book offers the lay reader a rare glimpse of the world on the other side of the stethoscope."
— *The Journal of the American Medical Association*

"Timothy McCall is wonderful. He understands people, and better still, he cares. Examining Your Doctor enables you to avoid the traps that lurk every time you visit the doctor. The drug chapter alone is worth the price of admission. Don't leave home without it."
— Joe Graedon,
   author of *The People's Pharmacy*

"Whether for ferreting out questionable medical practices or deepening respect for individual practitioners, this is an engaging and useful resource."
— *Booklist*

"This is the rare book endorsed both by mainstream authorities and by health care activists."
— *The Detroit Free Press*

NB: Due to the publisher's bankruptcy, this book is long-since out of print. Subscribers to Timothy's email newsletter, however, will receive a free copy of the chapter, "Is Your Doctor Prescribing the Right Drugs?" http://www.drmccall.com/subscribe.html

"Dr. McCall provides a much needed service to all patients who find themselves in need of conventional medical care…Given the uncertainties and dangers of modern medicine, this is a most useful guide for patients and families."

— Andrew Weil, MD,
   University of Arizona College of Medicine,
   author of *Spontaneous Healing*

"The surprising thing to me about "Examining Your Doctor" was how readable it is…a book to be kept and reread."

— *The Atlanta Journal Constitution*

"An easy-to-read, sophisticated discussion of how to judge the quality of your medical care and get what's best for you. Highly recommended for doctors as well as patients."

— Richard Feinbloom, MD,
   Former Director, Family Health Care
   Program, Harvard Medical School

"One of our best finds… very informative and accessible."

— The National Women's
   Health Network

"McCall's book is meant to help patients expect—and get—the very best from their physicians, even in these days of impersonal HMOs and shrinking medical choices."

— *The Philadelphia Inquirer*

"A means to balance the often lopsided power equation of patient and physician."

— *Publishers Weekly*

"The ultimate guide in taking control of your medical care, this is truly a book that will pay for itself over and over."

— *Newsday*

YOGA AS MEDICINE®
SEMINARS AND TEACHER TRAININGS

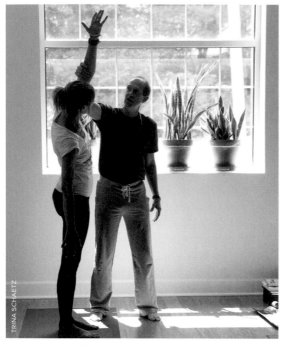

Periodically, Timothy teaches seminars on yoga therapy in various locations around the world. His flagship course is a 5-day, 30-hour, hands-on, roll-up-your-sleeves training called Yoga As Medicine (YAM), Level 1. It is recommended for yoga students, yoga teachers and aspiring yoga therapists, as well as health care professionals and holistic healers. He also teaches more advanced YAM seminars as well as courses in what he calls "holistic yoga anatomy."

For more information and a schedule of upcoming offerings, please see DrMcCall.com, or sign up for Dr. Timothy's free email newsletter.

www.drmccall.com/yoga-as-medicine-level-1.html

http://www.drmccall.com/subscribe.html